SUPPORTING PATIENTS LIVING WITH DEMENTIA DURING A PANDEMIC

Nicola Abraham and
Ma. Victoria Ruddock

SUPPORTING PATIENTS LIVING WITH DEMENTIA DURING A PANDEMIC

Digital theatre and educational spaces

The Education Studies Collection

Collection Editor
Janise Hurtig

First published in 2022 by Lived Places Publishing

The authors and editors have made every effort to ensure the accuracy of information contained in this publication, but assumes no responsibility for any errors, inaccuracies, inconsistencies and omissions. Likewise, every effort has been made to contact copyright holders. If any copyright material has been reproduced unwittingly and without permission the Publisher will gladly receive information enabling them to rectify any error or omission in subsequent editions.

British Library Cataloguing in Publication Data
A CIP record for this book is available from the British Library

ISBN: 9781915271037 (pbk)
ISBN: 9781915271044 (ePDF)
ISBN: 9781915271051 (ePUB)

The right of Nicola Abraham and Ma. Victoria Ruddock to be identified as the Authors of this work have been asserted by her in accordance with the Copyright, Design and Patents Act 1988.

Cover design by Fiachra McCarthy
Book design by Rachel Trolove of Twin Trail Design
Typeset by Newgen Publishing UK

Lived Places Publishing
Long Island
New York 11789

www.livedplacespublishing.com

For the students, patients and NHS staff who have worked with us on this journey and the friends and family who have supported us, we would like to say a huge thank you for your creativity, playfulness and collaboration.

Abstract

This book tells the story of how digital applied theatre was adapted to support patients living with dementia across hospitals in a pandemic. The challenges, successes and opportunities that this unusual project, Innovating Knowledge Exchange, created are shared in this book that acts as a guide to person-centred online practice. The narratives of the book share insights into horizontal team structures as ways of supporting students learning this evolving practice that adapted to COVID-19 restrictions and in doing so opened up a whole new world of possibilities for creative practice to support the wellbeing of older adult patients in acute hospital contexts. We hope you find the journey of the evolution of this new type of practice as useful and exciting to read as we have to live, dream and advance.

Keywords

Dementia; healthcare; higher education; applied theatre; practical experience; stories; students; virtual learning; pedagogy; education studies.

Notes on contributors

Dr Nicola Abraham

Senior Lecturer in Applied Theatre Practices at the Royal Central School of Speech and Drama. She has most recently been working on a range of applied theatre, film and virtual reality (VR) projects in NHS hospitals to develop new person-centred approaches to creating bespoke artefacts, including: VR360 videos; intergenerational augmented reality-based process dramas with primary school children and older adult patients living with dementia; and films to improve the subjective wellbeing of patients in acute dialysis wards. She has published in *Research in Drama Education: The Journal of Applied Theatre and Performance* (*RiDE*), *Applied Theatre Research*, *Contemporary Theatre Review*, *English Teachers Association Switzerland* and *Welfare e Ergonomia*, and co-edited the second edition of *The Applied Theatre Reader* (2020) and *Applied Theatre with Urban Youth: Witnessing Change* (forthcoming, 2023).

Ma. Victoria Ruddock

Dementia Specialist Healthcare Support Worker for the Dementia Care Team within Imperial College Healthcare NHS Trust, seconded to Co-Project Lead of the collaborative Innovating Knowledge Exchange project in partnership with the Royal Central School of Speech and Drama. She has a Bachelor of

Science degree in Nursing from the Philippines and has extensive experience working with older adults living with dementia and experiencing delirium in both hospitals and care home contexts. Victoria has additionally undertaken team leadership support in a nursing home and work as a private nurse for people living with dementia. Victoria has also taken part in a TEDx talk about her work facilitating applied theatre projects in acute dialysis wards and Medicine for the Elderly wards with students.

Contents

Acknowledgements

We would like to thank Jo James for her inspirational "say yes" approach to collaboration and the Office for Students and Research England for funding our work.

Learning objectives

This book addresses the following five learning objectives. The aim is to enable readers to step into the shoes of the practitioners who have worked with us, across disciplines, in order to learn about dementia and applied theatre in care contexts.

Objective one

- To engage readers in a journey of discovery through vignettes of project experiences to help support understanding about the ways in which facilitators can work responsively online in acute hospital settings with patients living with dementia.

Objective two

- To offer insights into best practice working digitally within arts and health hospital contexts.

Objective three

- To provide suggested assignments to support students' learning and development as community arts and health practitioners creating practice to improve wellbeing.

Objective four

- To develop readers' understanding of the importance of reciprocity in digital applied theatre projects to avoid extractive ways of working that aren't as dementia-friendly as they could be.

Objective five

- To think about how we navigate social identities in digital spaces to build connections through creativity.

Introduction

We begin our tale in the middle of a global pandemic. We locate our story in acute hospitals within Medicine for the Elderly wards in London, UK, working with people living with dementia through digital applied theatre projects. We have two main characters in this tale: Vic, a dementia specialist healthcare support worker, and Nicky a senior lecturer in applied theatre Practices. This may sound like an odd pairing to you, but for us the projects we discuss and the journey we share in this book are the culmination of five years of collaborative projects between applied theatre practitioners and a dementia care team who work within one of the biggest hospital trusts in the United Kingdom, Imperial College Healthcare NHS Trust. With funding from Research England and the Office for Students, we were able to more than quadruple the number of projects we offered to creatively engage with patients living with dementia in hospital wards.

The pandemic and lockdown hit in March 2020, which could have thrown our plans to upscale our in-person work into disarray. However, as a partnership, we are dedicated to innovation; our one rule for working together is to "say yes" to ideas and discover ways to make our ideas a reality. We decided to continue with our plans despite the pandemic for this reason, and for the added reason that the urgent need to support patients living with dementia only increased in the pandemic. This is because of the change in rules in hospitals and care homes that meant visitors were no longer allowed to see their relatives in person.

The impact of COVID-19 and long hospital stays has been detrimental for the wellbeing of patients and care home residents across the board, but particularly for people living with dementia. The projects we will discuss in this book are the result of collaborations between clinical specialist nurses; Jo James, consultant nurse in dementia and delirium and head of the dementia care team; and applied theatre practitioners working and studying in a drama school. Each project locates the patients who take part as artists at the heart of the work. There are six main projects that we make reference to as case study examples of practice in action. The projects are summarised below for context.

Auchi Street

This is a collaborative film-making project that is facilitated with patients living with dementia and/or undergoing dialysis. The project creates a collective fictional narrative, which patients then help to script, cast, direct or perform. The project team of applied theatre practitioners then film and edit the piece to premiere on the ward for patients, staff, family and friends.

Wonder VR

This is a project that usually happens one-to-one through a workshop that engages patients in creative tasks that explore places they like or would like to see. The stories are transformed into VR360 video experiences that students film and edit to present back to patients, in order to bring to life their stories as an immersive experience. This can help to transport a patient to a place they miss, would like to see or have invented.

Life in Lyrics

This is a song-writing project that works one-to-one with patients living with dementia to engage in experiences of music. The project is about sharing our love of music, singing along to our favourite songs, thinking about how we feel about music and forming ideas for an original song that is then co-written with patients, recorded and transferred to CD.

Hear Me Out

This is a podcasting project that connects family, friends and patients in hospital. It is a storytelling project that shares recollections, current thinking and future dreams and often involves recordings from siblings and children. Recordings are then edited into one podcast that all parties can listen to, to hear one another's voices as a form of celebration of life stories and as a comfort when families are unable to be together because of the pandemic.

Intergen

This is an intergenerational project that connects school children with patients living with dementia. The project has many models depending on the collaborative partners at the time and has involved collaborative storytelling, solving mysteries together and sharing stories of inspiration between patients and children/young people.

Your Story Your Way

This project asks participants to think about stories that communicate an aspiration or cherished experience, explored through a creative workshop. The participants can then ask for their story to be represented in any way they wish. For example, we have had requests for audiobooks, animations, puppets, paintings, radio shows, music videos, poems and performances, to name but a few.

Digital applied theatre

The term "digital applied theatre practice" underpins our values, ethics and the creative approach to all of our projects. So what exactly do we mean by this phrase? Applied theatre is an umbrella term that has been used to describe a set of practices that have similar traits. For example, often practices under this umbrella are focused around making theatre with, by and for communities (Prentki and Preston, 2009). Applied theatre practices are also concerned with participation, socio-political contexts, responsive cultural practice, development, challenging oppression and advocating for social changes; applied theatre means to use theatre as a tool to address these themes. The practices under the umbrella of applied theatre take place in a range of contexts including schools, prisons, hospitals, care homes, refugee centres, detention centres, community centres and on the streets. Practices working with communities are sensitive to cultural differences and seek to understand the interests, circumstances and context of the communities that they engage with to avoid neo-colonial models of practice that assume superiority of Western values and middle-class sentiments. Being open and responsive are core qualities inherent in applied theatre practices, and questioning the ethics of different approaches is the subject of much debate and ongoing critical thinking to help advance the field to continue being politically aware and engaged and to model best practice (Kerr, 2009). Applied theatre practice is responsive to the needs of the community and not only requires practitioners in this field to be artists leading participants as co-artists, but also seeks to be supportive of participants as a communi:y. Kay Hepplewhite (2021) offers a useful summary of responsivity in applied theatre practice.

> Responsivity foregrounds the participants as an ethical proposition. The practitioner operates at their most *responsive* when they are aware of the participants' experiences and how they can enable potential outcomes. However, the practitioners' own *response* and being open to development is also a key component of their expertise; they share a focus on impact and change.
>
> (2021: 4)

Hepplewhite's discussion of responsivity in applied theatre also brings to light how important it is for applied theatre practitioners to be open and adaptable to the needs and context of the community they are working with. This is a key priority for our practice with patients living with dementia to ensure that we offer person-centred practice that locates the participant as artist at the heart of our work. The second point that Hepplewhite raises concerns the priorities of applied theatre practitioners, which are often bound by funding agendas that prioritise a focus on the economic and social benefit of applied theatre in different contexts (see social prescription, Calderón-Larrañaga et al., 2021). This can be a competing demand when trying to locate the value in applied theatre practice because we also have to balance the impact that participants themselves locate in the projects that they take part in, and these can clash with or not register on funding impact assessment indicators.

A further issue within the field that warrants discussion is the focus on change as a measure of worth. Kelly Freebody et al. (2018: 6) detail the challenges of understanding what constitutes, and what is meant by, change in applied theatre, placing caution on practices that "see the world through its problems worth fixing". This framing raises questions about whether practitioners approaching applied theatre are seeing their participants "from a deficit perspective" (2018: 6) and seeing communities as a problem to fix. This is arguably the very neo-colonial power imbalance we want to avoid in applied theatre practice. For this reason, it's certainly a perspective that we do not follow in our projects, because we want to *challenge* stigma and prejudiced perceptions of people living with dementia rather than feeding into that stigma. In our practice, we start from a position of viewing the participant as an artist, and we agree that it is part of the creative process to find the most accessible and inclusive routes to working with each individual to celebrate identity and value the ideas that we have the privilege of learning from our participants.

Finding ways for applied theatre practice to support people living with dementia is important. Sheila McCormick (2017) discusses the role of the arts as an alternative model of intervention that can support people living with dementia by offering cognitive stimulation, social interaction and communication to improve quality of life. McCormick argues that creative arts offer an opportunity for positive connection for people living with dementia and practitioners.

> Looking to creative approaches to meeting the needs of people with dementia has helped to support people to continue to live well in their community through fostering connections and meeting the needs of individuals through the arts at what can be a challenging time for anyone affected by dementia.
>
> (2017: 227)

In this reading of the impact of arts for people living with dementia it is clear that there is a need for meaningful activities which embody the qualities of responsive practice and are adaptable and enjoyable for participants. In adapting our practice for the pandemic, it was important that our model of applied theatre practice maintained the same values that we had in-person within our new digital practice. Practically speaking, this looks like applied theatre workshops in song-writing, film-making, storytelling and podcasting that have been facilitated partly over Zoom by student practitioners and supported by specialists in dementia and navigating clinical environments and a specialist in applied theatre and technology. For us, digital tools have opened up a new type of practice in applied theatre, one that patients have experienced as less invasive than in-person work. They have also allowed us to transcend the limits of social restrictions to connect with care homes, schools and hospitals around London safely at a time when the need for creative engagement and social interaction has increased. This book charts what we have learnt from the process of translating applied theatre practice in person to an online digital practice that continues to embody the values of person-centred practice.

Sharing stories

In this book, we have placed a strong emphasis on honesty and transparency as a way to articulate and share our learning by drawing upon our own experience. You will see our names in brackets when we change authorial voice to signal whose story you are hearing at different points in the text, like this: **[Vic]** or **[Nicky]** or **[Both]**. Experience and personal narrative are woven into the fabric of each chapter, and we invite readers to reflect and add their own stories to the tapestry of stories that we have offered.

Both of us value learning from, with and within our teams of students, and from and with our participants. To do this, we need to understand one another's positions and reasons for taking part in the field. In the next section, we offer a first glimpse of our practice of sharing by charting our personal journeys and interests in working in the arts and health as an evolving field of practice.

Vic's story

[Vic] Since I was little, I knew I was different from other kids my age. I used to love to sing and dance; I started singing when I was three years old, and my dad encouraged me to pursue this interest. I learnt to sing even before I learnt to read; my Dad used to dictate the lyrics of my favourite songs to me, and I learnt them by heart before recording them on a multiplex cassette tape with my sister. We would then send the cassette tape to my mum, who was working overseas as a charge nurse in a dialysis unit. These tapes were my musical letters to my mum, to let her know that I loved her, and I thoroughly enjoyed the process of learning and making her these gifts, knowing the joy they would bring her. I started singing as a member of our community choir a few years later. As a child, I preferred spending time with older adults in my family rather than playing with other children my age. I remember always feeling fascinated listening to the conversations between my grandparents and enjoyed looking at their facial expressions while they were talking with each other – they were always animated storytellers and I enjoyed and have taken on these traits myself.

I should also mention that I grew up with my grandparents, so they were very close to me, especially my nan, who passed away with dementia. Because of her, I was inspired to work with older adults, especially people living with dementia. It was partly as a tribute to my nan, but also to make sure people living with dementia feel valued and heard – both important things for good quality of life. My devotion and passion were amplified further when I started my nursing degree for my bachelor of science in the Philippines, where I was born.

I have always seen a synergy between arts and health, and I continued to find ways to pursue both interests while I was at college. For example, while I was training to be a nurse, I was also a member of a university-based theatre company called "Tiatro", which means "theatre". In Tiatro, I was the assistant choreographer and a singer who, on behalf of my college, represented the school at local competitions. I also taught other members of the theatre group dance choreography that was a combination of street dance and modern dance. I really enjoyed the feeling that you get when you perform, and the excitement of creating something from scratch. Learning about performance at the same time as studying nursing, I could see a natural connection evolving between both fields, particularly in the way that the arts could be used to improve wellbeing.

As a result of this life experience during my college years, I developed a strong interest in the purpose of the arts in clinical settings. I always asked myself, *how am I going to incorporate arts into healthcare now I can see the potential of the arts to improve wellbeing?* I wasn't expecting that during my career within Imperial College Healthcare NHS (National Health Service) Trust this opportunity would arise. Before I worked with Nicky, I worked in Medicine for the Elderly wards as a dementia specialist healthcare support worker in a dementia care team in London, UK and tried my best to bring the arts into my practice. For example, while my patients were eating their breakfast, I sang to them, and they greatly appreciated and enjoyed this experience. I would even take requests, asking patients for song preferences and ideas!

What also touched my heart is that even though the patients were very poorly and in pain, when they heard music, their facial expressions changed, and they enjoyed singing along with me. Even though sometimes we'd be singing our own versions of the songs, it didn't matter; what mattered was that they appreciated what I did for them. That inspired me to continue to sing for my patients every day during breakfast time. I hadn't realised that someone had witnessed what I'd done to make patients' experience better in hospitals, but I soon found that my line manager at the time was amazed by the impact of this gesture of creative kindness. My approach was also acknowledged by broader patient specialist teams in the Trust, which encouraged me further to use my imagination, passion and creativity to improve patient care.

In July 2021, Imperial launched a gratitude festival for NHS staff and one of the events was *Imperial's Got Talent*, calling upon staff across the Trust to submit acts to be judged by leaders in Imperial. Our act was a collaborative song called *Have a Little Faith* (Abraham, 2021a), which was performed by staff from a Medicine for the Elderly ward in addition to staff from the dementia care team. I sang the lead vocal, and Nicky and her dad wrote the music and lyrics. Little did we know that our submission would reach the grand final, where it was judged by Elton John and David Furnish and awarded first place. This recognition meant a lot to the staff, and allowed us to celebrate the collective artistic talents of NHS staff. The competition represented yet another way to integrate the arts into healthcare.

I was excited to be given the opportunity to work on the Innovating Knowledge Exchange project with Nicky, which is a digital applied theatre project in acute hospital settings, because I hadn't realised arts and health could be connected in so many ways. The impact of this combination is huge for patient wellbeing and improves patient health through positive creative engagement. This type of cognitively stimulating interaction helps patients to feel more alert, more positive and more valued during their stay.

You would also be shocked to learn how many patients are also artists and share a passion for creativity. It always amazes me how having a patient who holds the same passion as you makes work in the hospital easier, because of the innate connection that naturally evolves. With this connection, you build rapport with one another and build trust in the process. Part of my work embodies person-centred practice, which happens in creative exchanges. Working with creative collaborative partnerships to offer bespoke, engaging workshops makes a significant difference to the lives of our patients while they are in hospital or in care homes. I have learnt that by incorporating my artistic knowledge with my medical knowledge in my own way, I can inspire others and improve the wellbeing and experience of the people in hospital who I have the privilege of working with. My advice to those interested in arts and health is to embrace your imagination, share your talents, apply them to different contexts and to not be afraid to try, offer, revise and advance your practice – that's how you change the world.

My focal point of inspiration is my patients and a simple thank you from them means a lot to me and inspires me to push myself to do more for them. This is why I am paying this lesson forward to you in the hope that you will continue to inspire others. I would like to task you with passing forward your passion and talents too. It just goes to show that what you do can make a difference.

Nicky's story

[Nicky] My journey into arts and health started with a situation I faced in my teenage years that inspired me to understand how theatre could make a difference to the lives of communities. It began when I was around 13 years old; my parents had divorced, and at that point this wasn't really heard of in my community. There were some "friends" who turned their backs on me, and others who just didn't know what to say. For respite, I would go to a youth club in my hometown. It had a tuck shop, a sports hall and a small theatre space with a stage and a wooden DJ box. The theatre was often occupied by the kids I was a bit scared of; they were popular and had a reputation of "don't mess with me". I would spend time with a close group of friends playing basketball and talking to the lady who ran the tuck shop. She must have been in her mid-eighties, and she loved children. She always made us feel welcome and liked to sit and chat to us about life, ambitions and our interests. We adored this lady, and she was a big part of our experience in the youth centre – and, clearly, interacting with children and young people held equal value for her. Then one day we came in and the youth leader who was in charge sat us down and said they were losing funding and would have to close. This was devastating news to all of us, and I remember thinking: I really can't lose this place, rough around the edges though it is, it's too important, because it's just ours for this time once a week and it makes all the difference.

I gathered my friends, who were all worried too, and said what can we do, and what do we have? I had a slightly scratched karaoke CD in my bag, and they had ideas for a script that could unite the songs. We sketched out a plan but needed to use the theatre, so we had to be brave and talk to the kids who owned that space to seek their help – not something I was looking forward to then. remember taking a deep breath, walking into the hall, my friends in a line close behind me, looking a little terrified about what we were about to do. I was told to leave the second I entered the room, but I held firm, heart pounding in my chest, and explained in brief what was going to happen to the youth club and that we had a plan to raise money to save it. After ducking a few flying shoes that were poorly aimed at my head, the group dispersed and, to our amazement, many people stayed to help us.

It was certainly not an easy process; there were walk-outs, strops, tantrums and disagreements. But there was also a lot of laughter, new friendships and a strong unified need to make this plan a success. After a month of rehearsing at school, and in the youth club, we'd devised a one-hour show complete with post-show karaoke and invited everyone we knew. I remember waiting behind the dusty stage curtains and being so nervous I thought I might be sick, but fortunately I wasn't! We all had everything crossed in the hope people would actually show up. Walking on stage to start, I wanted to cry; the auditorium was packed full of people – familiar faces, new faces, teachers, friends, relatives, neighbours, community members we'd never met and local press had come to cover the show and support us. We did our best, and though I'm sure it wasn't anywhere near the quality of a professional show, it got a lot of laughs, and people sang along, and we raised hundreds of pounds and saved the youth club.

I remember thinking at that time how much better and stronger I felt being with a community, albeit a dysfunctional one at times, to achieve something together. That feeling still stays with me every time I start a new academic year with my students. I decided, after that show, to spend my life understanding how we got past our differences and fought for what we believed in, and how we could give that feeling to other people. I hope my students will benefit from what I have understood and do the same for their communities in their practices.

The opportunity to work with older adults in a clinical context arrived in 2016. I'd achieved my PhD researching impact and change in applied theatre for young people, and was in my second year as a lecturer in applied theatre practices. A rogue e-mail meant for someone else arrived for me from our reception team, who thought I may be able to help. A hospital in London had sent an e-mail asking if drama schools could offer some theatre to put on for patients in Medicine for the Elderly wards. I was intrigued by this idea and thought of my work with people living with dementia from previous projects, and community activist groups run by older adults, and how much I learnt and loved working with both groups. I replied straight away and met with Jo, a consultant nurse in dementia and delirium from the dementia care team, and her colleague, a healthcare support worker from the same NHS trust. I explained in that first meeting that we could of course create theatre *for* patients but wondered how they felt about making theatre *with* patients, explaining that applied theatre locates participants at the heart of the practice. We devised our first project, working in two-week cycles to deliver in-person workshops in day rooms on wards for patients living with dementia. This happened through a series of workshops, held over two weeks and culminated in a participatory performance devised with patients, which repeated three times. Following the success of this project, we were then challenged by Jo and her team to create an interactive project for older adults undergoing dialysis treatment and created Auchi Street – a collaborative film-making project, working bed-to-bed and involving patients in the creation of everything from narrative to casting, scripting and set design.

At the same time as this project, I developed an interest in learning how to make VR360 films as immersive experiences, and proposed to Jo an idea for a project called Wonder VR to offer patients in long-term hospital care a way to see the places they missed. We have created over 40 films now for patients. This project became the most popular one we offered during the pandemic, with people staying longer in hospital when they caught COVID, and missing places that were part of their daily routine. The more projects we created, the more we realised that there were increased opportunities, possibilities and a need for more interventions on a more regular basis. Jo and Imperial Health Charity, a charity attached to the trust we worked with, created a fellowship project. This idea had a junior doctor taking charge of an intergenerational project, which she asked me to help deliver. We offered training workshops in dementia and communication through drama in schools and sessions for patients and children; this combined my previous and my current research and ignited a strong desire in me to recreate the connections I felt with the lady in the tuck shop all those years ago for the young people I was encountering. I knew both age groups could bring joy to each other, so I was delighted to bring my students to join me in facilitating a range of workshops over two years for the Intergen project.

In December 2019, there was an opportunity to apply for a joint bid for Knowledge Exchange funding from Research England and the Office for Students, which would enable us to deliver projects all year round to all wards in the trust. This would also enable us to upscale our training for students by the dementia care team and I, by both sharing our experience and guiding them through live practice on various projects. We weren't deterred by the pandemic, having already had to make 15 collaborative projects happen in digital form for our second-year students when lockdown hit the UK in the spring and summer terms of 2020. Jo took a leap of faith and allowed me to learn and adapt, and continue to grow our work online, with students joining and learning via Zoom while Vic and I, alongside other members of the dementia care team, supported patients in person. We engaged students in developing more projects with us, including a project on music called Life in Lyrics, a podcast called Hear Me Out and a project celebrating patient stories called Your Story Your Way. When the opportunity came to share our knowledge of online practice and versions of our work, we jumped at the chance to write down and share what we have learnt over the past two years with you, in the hope that you will support older adults living with dementia and see the urgency of practice in this field online. We are fortunate to have safe online practice available to us; a decade ago, I think we would have struggled to support older adults, and now we have learnt that online practice is both less invasive and more creative and playful as a COVID-safe way to continue offering meaningful interactions for patients and residents living with dementia.

What will your story be?

We're excited to take you on this journey of discovery with us. We hope that you seek opportunities to collaborate and offer your skills, artistry, care and support for partnerships with other educational and healthcare contexts, and that our guidance is useful. We also advise you to always seek guidance from experts you are working with and to follow their rules, regulations, precautions and advice at all times. This has been vital for our practice. We also know that advice and guidance changes as research develops and grows, so we advise you to keep up to date with training and learning in this field, and to work with expert partners to ensure you offer best practice. This book maps the things we have learnt that we hope you find useful, but what we did is just one path and way of working. What follows enabled us to deliver bespoke creative practice for people living with dementia during a global pandemic; we hope it helps you as you develop your own stories.

1

Acute ambitions to be yourself (I)

There are several points throughout this chapter, and the rest of the book, where we will ask you to reflect on your own experience in relation to examples from our practice. Please do take the time to pause and reflect. Being reflective is important to ensure that we are "thinking practitioners", who consider their actions and the implications of their choices in practice. This is a way to "check in" on our intentions as practitioners, to ensure that we are considering the ethics of our choices and taking an empathetic approach to our practice.

Considering who we are and why we are

You have most likely experienced a situation or conversation, at some point in your life, in which the person you are talking to does not "get you". Perhaps if it is a small, ill-informed but well-intentioned comment this may make you feel slightly irritated, or it may be a more cutting and upsetting comment, especially if it is witnessed by others who have agreed with the misreading of your identity. People misunderstanding who you are, what you stand for and what holds meaning for you is not a pleasant experience. Now, imagine that before you walked into this conversation, you had felt disempowered and not listened to for the *entire day* preceding this interaction. Imagine that you have been trying to challenge these hurtful perceptions about you, but that you can't quite find the pause in the conversation to intervene, nor is anyone really hearing what you are saying when you do interject. Think of this encounter, and how it may make you feel. Ask yourself the following questions to unpack your thoughts.

Reflect

1.   **What emotion(s) are you feeling?**
2.   **What is it like feeling this way?**
3.   **How does this feeling affect your day?**
4.   **Does this change your mood for a moment, or does it stay with you?**

Our identities are necessarily complex. They are formed and informed by many factors: by our genetics, the way we interact with the world, the way the world constructs its view of us and our experiences. Identity is not a simple concept to distil into a sentence; we are complicated and proud of this. Our humanity is bound in our complexity, and the events in our life that have informed our identity and self-perception are important parts of who we are. When we feel misunderstood, overlooked, forgotten or unheard, we feel that our identity has been distorted and misrepresented by those who perform these behaviours. It hurts us when people underestimate our abilities, it frustrates us when we feel no one places value upon what we contribute to the world and it is painful to feel forgotten or as if our existence doesn't matter.

These ideas about identity may sound far-fetched or may be overly dramatic to you. If so, then you are lucky to never have been in a position of feeling powerless. To understand this further, let us pause for a moment and consider the relationship between being misunderstood and models of power. Jo Rowlands (2008) offers useful insights into models of power that help us to understand how power may manifest negatively. Rowlands' definition of "power over" is the model that offers most concern for us within our practice. There have been numerous studies that contest the way power has been asserted over people living with dementia, within their care and within the assumptions made about communication of their wants and needs in their everyday lives. Being in a vulnerable position – for example, not easily being able to state your opinion or respond to questions – is frustrating, and often leads others to speak over and for you. This is a type of "power over"; it is an action that takes away your choice and chance to state your own response or preference. Power over is a negative model of power, one that takes away autonomy and consequently dehumanises you. We found that it is essential, when working with people who might struggle to articulate choices in clear speech, that we find alternative ways to communicate when offering responsive creative practice. We need ways to communicate that don't rely on or prioritise speech, and instead seek to embrace a way of understanding an individual through learning about them and offering creative avenues to inclusion. For example, this may involve presenting options a participant can point to using symbols or speaking to family and friends to learn someone's interests, which are then incorporated into workshops to engage a patient in something they like. This avoids power over models of working that *assume* rather than discover or ask what is important to a person living with dementia.

The consequences of taking a power over approach are further elaborated on by Tom Kitwood. Patients living with dementia who have experienced being talked about or over are regularly confronted with false and negative constructs about themselves. These are constructs that Tom Kitwood (1997) terms malignant social psychology (MSP). Kitwood is an advocate for personhood and person-centred care that values the individual experiences, needs, journey and identity of each individual living with dementia. He describes/defines MSP as both an active and passive (neglect) marginalising way of interacting with people living with dementia. Kitwood lists the following elements of MSP.

> […] treachery […] disempowerment […] infantilization
> […] intimidation […] labelling […] stigmatization
> […] outpacing […] invalidation […] banishment
> […] objectification […] ignoring […] imposition
> […] withholding […] accusation […] disruption […]
> mockery […] disparagement
>
> (Kitwood, 1997: 46–47)

Each element demonstrates a lack of care, a lack of acknowledgement of human rights and a lack of acknowledgement of individual identity or personhood for people living with dementia. It is also important to consider the implications of MSP on anxiety levels for people living with dementia, both at home and in care homes, if this is the type of care they receive. Kitwood elaborates, stating that "Malignancy tends to increase in proportion to three factors: fear, anonymity and the differential of power" (1997: 48). Fear is a complex emotion and one that causes much unrest for patients and care home residents alike. It can present as being afraid to speak out because you may be mocked or infantilised; fear may keep people from asking for help or medication n case they are not heard. Or people may feel there is little point requesting support when the response is uncaring or negative. This neglectful state of affairs, of course, is not always the case for people living with dementia in care homes, at home or in hospital, but there are many cases where MSP sadly persists. In our approach to working with people living with dementia, then, we must not replicate these kinds of dehumanising practices. Instead, we must find ways throughout all our work to offer counter-narratives and experiences that celebrate personhood, and that value individuals for their experience. Let's now explore the ways in which we have adapted our digital applied theatre practice to work in a way that is responsive to the needs, ideas and creativity of people living with dementia.

Virtual practice

It has been our ambition for the digital applied theatre versions of our projects to ensure we offer unapologetically "bespoke" (a term that we are using to describe individual and personalised interactions and/or artefacts; see Glossary) and meaningful workshops that are tailored to the needs, ideas and personal experiences of each individual participant. To ensure we are following person-centred practice, we need to offer interactive and reciprocal practice that places value on the patients we work with through their engagement with our students. When it works, patients are excited and find wonder in the interactions they experience, and students reflect their delight at patient responses; however, achieving this level of connection over online media isn't easy. The journey to achieve effective practice that offers high-quality interactions is complex. It requires student facilitators to sit comfortably with the many types of uncertainty that inform and are necessarily part of the context of working in a ward. Machines are beeping; crash teams are on stand-by; nurses are taking observational notes, checking blood pressure and taking COVID swabs; porters are moving patients for scans or transport. Wards are busy places. They are full of a myriad of clinicians working hard to help people recover from different types of illness or injuries. Working in this environment is difficult at points. However, it is necessary if we are to bring applied theatre to the people who need it; people on a ward may need to engage with cognitively stimulating activities that inspire hope, especially in the bleakest of times. This isn't just practice that offers momentary interaction; its purpose runs much deeper.

Practice with purpose is about:

- supporting the wellbeing of older adults living with dementia;
- being inclusive, to support access to our workshops and adapt our approach to meet the needs of our participants;
- creating a sense of community in the loneliest of times for those in side rooms or without visitors;
- valuing ideas from a patient or care home resident living with dementia, and thereby valuing individual interests, talents and identity;

- seeing the patient as an artist at the heart of digital applied theatre practice;
- building intergenerational connection between people living with dementia and facilitators online in addition to in person clinical and non-clinical staff supporting projects;
- supporting the artistic vision and aspirations of participants;
- celebrating ideas and actively listening to participants by always saying "yes" to requests and finding ways to bring to fruition the suggestions given in sessions;
- reciprocity embedded into our interactions with participants to share and not be extractive in our practice.

Creating responsive practice is paramount to offering what Jo James et al. term "meaningful activity" (2017: 12). James measures the usefulness of a given activity by the happiness of the person who has engaged in an interactive task. She additionally notes the implications of creative engagement, suggesting that "[A]ctivity can mean that relationships between patients and staff are strengthened, which can in turn lead to reduction in anxiety and agitation, and quite possibly to some physical changes – sitting out of bed more, perhaps walking more, improving sleep patterns" (2017: 146). From this perspective, there are benefits to the wellbeing of a person living with dementia when they engage with meaningful activity that addresses the feelings of loneliness and isolation that can arise from being in a hospital or care home with few or no visitors. Interaction in this sense is meaningful when it offers respite from silence and creates an avenue to be seen and heard as a person. Jill Hayes (2011) extends this idea further, suggesting that a person living with dementia who engages in creative arts activities benefits in three different ways, because the creative arts are a "vehicle for self", a "relational bridge" and also "healing" (2011: 32–36).

We may know from our own experience that some feelings are beyond words. In those situations, the creative arts can offer a way to communicate that transcends the limits of words. The feeling of recognition we get when someone hears us and actively listens, watches or engages with a story that we have chosen to share, in the form that we have chosen to share it in, can be very powerful. Hayes argues that this is the case for everyone, including people living with dementia, who "still love to sing, to dance, to make[...] As energy and passion build, the interaction between people grows stronger. The arts create new possibilities for communication and appreciation" (2011: 33). What is of note here is Hayes' call for opportunities for engagement and participation, and the power that such activity can offer a person living with dementia. And it's not just being heard; think of the human connection that naturally comes with artistic engagement. There is a sense of belonging that can occur when we are creating together – another way in which communication can be fostered through the arts.

We can liken this sense of belonging to experiences of seeing friends and loved ones after the national lockdowns that have occurred during the COVID-19 pandemic. We greet friends with warmth, care and relief after a long absence, and reassert our own identity through interaction with those we love and who care for us. When we engage with people living with dementia, even if this is for the first time, it is important that we show this same care, compassion and appreciation for each individual. Hayes notes that "[R]elationships give us confirmation of who we are and give meaning to our lives. They affirm our identity, and they can affirm our inner life too[…] We are appreciated through the eyes of another, therefore we appreciate our own life" (2011: 33). However, this dynamic is complex; it's not a science so much as a subjective experience. This means not every relationship or interaction may have the level of impact suggested here; even though we are open and reciprocal in our creative exchanges, we must be wary of *expecting* the same in return. Instead, what we are doing is simply offering ideas to create a safe space for exchanges to happen over a tablet screen. When we do succeed in creating opportunities to be creative together, what we have learnt is that appreciation and reciprocity build similar or parallel feelings of affirmation through creativity and collaboration to those mentioned by Hayes (2011).

Delivering digital applied theatre workshops that offer creative opportunities, communications and outlets is important, not only for the impact of the workshops for patients, but also the intention and delivery of the practice. For example, if we say we are person-centred, and yet we offer workshops that are only one-sided and without reciprocity, we may well be seen as *extractive* in our practice. This means we are only *taking* and *listening* to stories without celebrating identity. One way of avoiding extractive practice is to work artefacts into your practice. We have found that creating bespoke artefacts is a good way of celebrating patient ideas; you are creating something together that takes both a digital and physical form, for example, a song played on YouTube but given to patients on a CD, along with lyrics and a letter of thanks. In some of our projects, a letter can be used to commemorate the stories that have been generously shared in workshops. What's important is that we try to provide an artefact that is in the format requested by the patient.

However, it is not just the methodology alone that is important for working in this context. It is also essential to have a team of students who share certain ideals and intentions. We have found, for example, that many of the applied theatre practitioners who have worked with us share particular qualities, which lend themselves to responsive approaches to practice.

Responsive facilitators tend to:

- trust their own intuition, and that of their colleagues, to read situations;
- demonstrate a strong ability to listen deeply and attentively;
- have a genuine interest in storytelling and sharing ideas;
- express an innate drive to care for those they work with;
- embody a passion for collaboration and artistry;
- share a political ambition to change situations that are detrimental to their participants;
- offer workshops that embody a strong sense of support, with low structure, to follow the ideas and needs of the participant(s);
- exude an openness to learn, adapt to and respond to different communities and contexts.

These qualities represent a passion for equality, fairness, inclusion, access and adaptability – all of which are the responsibility of the responsive facilitator. It is the combination of these qualities that enables facilitators to ensure their practice holds participant autonomy as a core value and practice offer. Personalised practice that shows a clear drive to understand and respond to the individual needs of participants enables facilitators to provide bespoke workshops and resulting artefacts. NHS (National Health Service) England advocates for the importance of autonomy for patients. This includes drawing upon skills and opportunities for interventions within the community that offer more holistic and individualised models of care.

> Personalised care means people have choice and control over the way their care is planned and delivered, based on "what matters" to them and their individual strengths, needs and preferences. This happens within a system that supports people to stay well for longer and makes the most of the expertise, capacity and potential of people, families, and communities in delivering better health and wellbeing outcomes and experiences.
>
> (NHS England, 2019: 6)

Though we are not referring to clinical care in our examples of practice, we are thinking about how to understand "what matters" most to people living with dementia, and how we can celebrate this creatively. We are also thinking about how we can be responsive to participants to ensure they feel heard and understood. We have invented strategies for engagement to ensure that autonomy and responsiveness are possible in our digital practice, and supported by our approach to delivering sessions.

Transmedia

We have named a strategy we often "transmedia". Transmedia has become an essential tool to deliver "smooth" workshops to participants living with dementia. It is an interesting term; it is usually used to describe a type of interactive story or media that transcends one type of media, or links one narrative or piece of information to another. Andy Lavender (2017) explores the connecting traits of the internet and theatre as a way of "transmediating", offering insights into the qualities of transmediated performances delivered online. The internet can offer an extension to theatrical spaces that is "durational, three-dimensional, and involving co-presence – in and through this newer medium of communication" (Lavender 2017: 342). If we consider traditional models of theatre as those with a stage at one end of a large room with an audience facing it, then perhaps the way digital space can be experienced as offering new ways of creating stories or involving audiences directly in the action. This could be through, for example, interactive digital platforms where audience members have to vote or make decisions. It could also be through interactive media, for example, Google Jamboards – virtual whiteboards that can be shared, where anyone with a link can post an idea.

Here, it is useful to think about the concepts of co-presence and liveness to explain how transmedia allows us to create meaningful activities and connections through digital applied theatre practice on Zoom. Lavender calls upon Lars Elleström (2013), who suggests that there is "source medium" and "target medium" in instances of transmediation – in other words, "it depicts a linear movement from one medium to another" (Lavender, 2017: 342). So, if the applied theatre workshops that facilitators have devised are the source medium, then our target medium is Zoom as a virtual space that we use to deliver workshops in digital form to our participants. Lavender describes the internet as a multimedial medium where users are creators, consumers and spectators of content. Describing the key traits of this digital realm, Lavender continues:

> […] the Internet's performance of conjunction through separateness; its layering of spaces; its emphasis on the networked connectedness of people as a feature of temporal presence (or being in the 'now'); it's invitation to absorption and a form of immersion; it's disposition to information and personal presentation.
>
> (2017: 344)

The qualities of internet engagement allow us to move beyond the limits of physical space through engaging with "virtual co-presence", by being online together through platforms such as Zoom. The virtual presence and connection we can have on Zoom means that wherever we are in the world, we can collaborate and work together as a team to be present in real time with our participants. We can respond, we can demonstrate active listening and we can interact. We can augment our images on screen with virtual backgrounds, filters and layered reality to bring an imaginative space into our interactions. If, for example, a participant we are working with shares their love of visiting a beach, we can, in a matter of seconds, change our screens to reflect their interest. We can instantly share the screen to play their favourite song to sing together; we can research and display images of the school they once attended or share Google Earth images of the street where they grew up.

The instantaneous response that is available from digital applied theatre workshops creates a sense of wonder and magic for our participants. They often respond with laughter, surprise and joy to see, hear or experience locations, sounds and stories that we can conjure through transmedia in an instant. On the surface, this appears to be a simple process. However, there are additional challenges that we need to navigate in order to offer a "smooth" workshop experience for participants. There are many moments when wards are noisy, sound isn't easily audible, internet connections fail or facilitators need support. Fortunately, we have a secondary tool in action in our workshops to navigate the complexity of "live" digital practice. We use the messaging service WhatsApp to communicate between teams, access additional media and sync technologies to "put people in the same virtual space", in addition to putting them "*in the same time*, in appearance and interconnection" (Lavender, 2017: 352).

Figure 1.1 provides an overview of a typical workshop that we would run for our intergenerational project online. The top level shows the two groups of online participants – in this case, students in a secondary school and their teacher working on Zoom, and the facilitators who run the session online and navigate between the school and the patient – and the in-person participants supported by the dementia care team. This group are clinical experts and support the facilitation team and patient to communicate. On the next level we have the device that allows us to collaborate between multiple physical locations to meet COVID safety measures in the hospital and keep everyone safe. The tablet we use connects us through Zoom; it's allowed by infection control because it limits physical contact and allows us to deliver workshops online safely. The last level is the recipient and participant of the online communication and

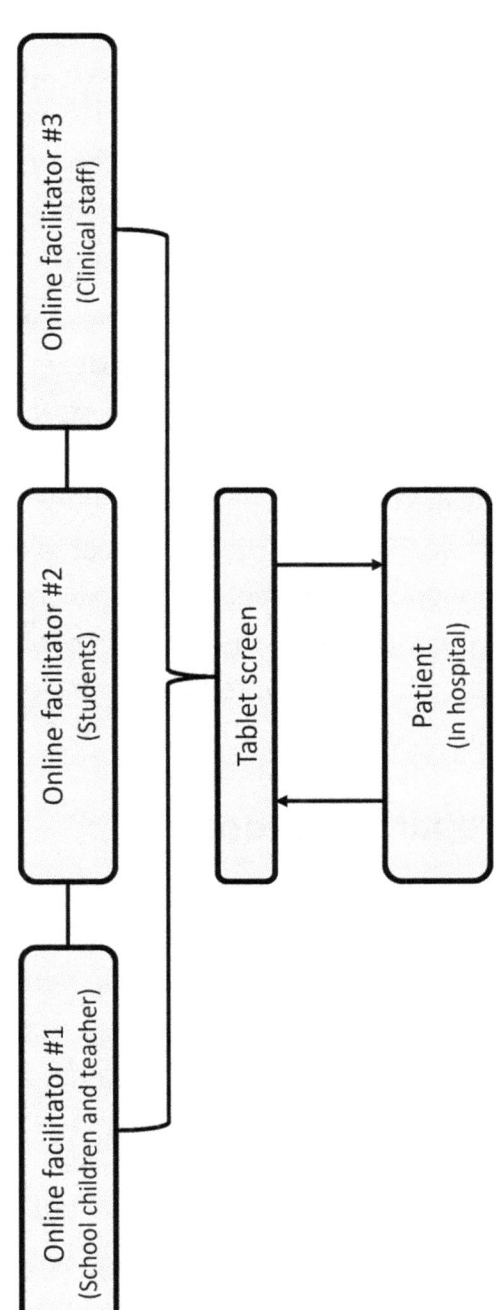

Figure 1.1 Summary transmedia communication diagram

workshop: the patient. Over the course of the pandemic, we have had various different configurations; for example, the school-based participants have at points been on individual screens, and at other points we have held hybrid practice through live classrooms and Zoom, or all being present in the classroom together.

Figure 1.2 illustrates a more detailed communication flow between the project team that includes the participant (patient), facilitators (students online) and in-person facilitation team (dementia care team staff). When we are using transmedia, it provides a route to connect the facilitators online with the in-person facilitation team to enable us to provide responsive facilitation approaches to support and engage the patient. Students facilitating can of course be in the same physical space, but they may also want to collaborate across the country or internationally to deliver workshops as a team.

Transmedia as a preparatory tool

Transmedia also allows us to support the team with preparatory information. A clinical member of staff will gather data from ward staff, who will identify which patients would most benefit from project interventions. As a clinical member of staff, the in-person facilitator #2 gathers information from the nurse in charge or ward manager to gain insights into patients who have been identified as having the capacity to participate. Once patients have been identified, the in-person clinical facilitator describes the project to the patient, and explains what it's about and how it happens, in order to support the patient to understand how they can interact with a tablet and students. If a patient consents,

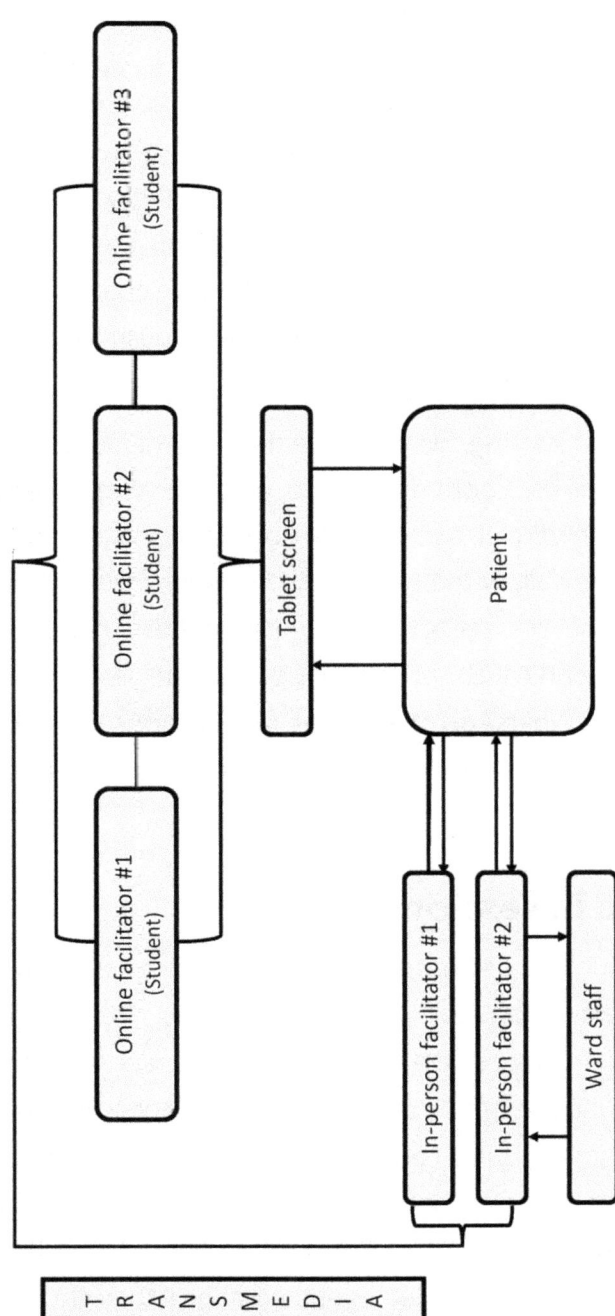

Figure 1.2 Transmedia information flow diagram

then the clinical facilitator disseminates their name, interests and any access needs to support – for example, visual or hearing impairments. They can also offer communication support strategies and advice to the online facilitation team ahead of the workshop. This is the first communication in preparation for the delivery of a one-off, one-to-one session, to support the patient in engaging with our projects. Students are then welcome to ask questions and gather information to clarify any questions they may have or ask for more support for adapting their ideas.

Prior to the session starting, we welcome the student facilitation team to the tablet on Zoom, to hand over co-hosting access. We refer to these digital access and hosting rights as their "superpowers"; they allow the team to share their screen, share sound and change any set-up options they need to for their workshop. Any technical issues that happen in the session are shared on a group WhatsApp chat, where all facilitators involved can provide live support, ask and answer questions and share resources.

Transmedia in sessions

During the session, we use transmedia to share pictures, found by the online facilitation team, that locate places the patient mentions. Sometimes these are conveyed using screen-sharing, but for patients who need more communication support we have found that this interruption can be disruptive and frustrating, whereas showing a photograph on a second device such as a phone is less intrusive and more exciting for the patient to see. This way, they can also zoom in on details of the image if they choose to. Taking this approach is great for allowing as many moments of autonomy as possible. Similarly, the facilitation group can also research favourite songs or genres of music to share with the patient; this can be done either on a tablet, showing lyrics on the screen, or as background music on an audio device. Since the response time using transmedia is incredibly fast, using music and images in this way can create great surprise and excitement.

Part of the role of the online facilitation team involves allocating responsibility to people for the different elements of a workshop. For example, someone will be responsible for researching and sharing YouTube links, photos and information to support the patient and demonstrate active listening. Another member of the team will then take responsibility for using sharing technologies to screen-share, sound-share or type information into Google Jamboards. The lead online facilitator can then use WhatsApp to transcend the screen and request material from their team, which allows them to focus on the screen to work with the patient. Should there be any issue with internet or sound, the team can also communicate this on WhatsApp. We advise everyone to have a co-pilot to smoothly hand over to in order to avoid jumpy calls for the patient; again, WhatsApp allows us to communicate this with ease. If there are problems for the team with hearing a softly spoken patient, or if there is a lot of noise on the ward, we also use transmedia to transcribe what the patient is saying, which helps to ease communication delays and avoid calls for the patient to repeat information, which can also be confusing or frustrating.

Overall, transmedia is an essential tool. We use this approach to ensure the patient has a seamless interaction with students online It allows us to demonstrate effective active listening through fast responses, screen-sharing, media-sharing and collaboration online. Transmedia also enables us to support the student team with timing, accessibility and any technical issues arising, to ensure that all participants feel calm throughout the session – even if there are unforeseen incidents on the ward. Transmedia additionally allows the in-person clinical facilitator to let the online team know about any changes in mood, or to identify if the patient is feeling tired or unwell in the session, which helps the team to know if we need to finish earlier than expected, or continue for longer than planned if the patient is enjoying the interaction. The teams are briefed about this possibility prior to projects commencing, and part of their training involves a reminder that patients are unwell and may suddenly feel worse and need rest. As part of best practice, we always follow clinical expertise and advice; transmedia allows us to communicate this instantaneously, which means we can always be responsive.

Examples and reflection

To understand how transmedia and a person-centred approach work to celebrate personhood in practice, two case studies follow.

Read through the examples carefully, and then think about your responses to the reflective questions at the end of each section. All names have been changed.

Case study #1 Jacob's story
Context

Working across hospital sites is challenging; you have to carry with you all the artefacts and technologies that you need for the day. But not only can it be physically heavy work; the logistics of arranging digital practice can weigh heavily on your mind, too. Travelling between hospitals, you find yourself thinking through the needs of your patients, the context of their stay in hospital and the requirements of your students on Zoom. You worry about the Wi-Fi and connections, and try to pre-empt what will happen in the session. You may harbour fear about whether a patient who consented to participate earlier in the day will still want to take part when you go to see them later. It's not unheard of for patient participants to drop out; reasons will vary, but it is often about pain, tiredness or feeling unwell and needing to rest, in addition to appointments, scans or visitors arriving unexpectedly. A sudden change of mind throws your careful preparation out the window. Suddenly, you need to think of a back-up plan to offer the workshop to another patient who will also benefit, but in this scenario you have significantly less time to prepare and must respond on the spot, employing your skills in spontaneity. We always manage to recruit another patient, as there are many who would benefit from the interventions we offer. But reflexively, it is a worry the project staff hold in their minds, and it is therefore essential that student facilitators on Zoom stay calm and ready to be responsive to support staff in these moments.

Jacob was a patient in a Medicine for the Elderly ward. He was referred to the project team to offer an intervention to support him, particularly around his engagement with staff. He wasn't coping with his situation very well at the time; in particular, he felt paranoid about what he was eating. Being in a side can also exacerbate feelings of loneliness; Jacob was feeling sad and upset, and staff reported that he was agitated and not settling on the ward, and paranoid about what was happening to him. He asked repeated questions to nursing staff about his food and because of his concern he didn't eat. His wife was there to support him with his eating to help him understand why he was admitted to the ward.

Before the session, we provided students with essential information through WhatsApp, to help them build connections with the patient. This often includes the patient's interests, hobbies, any access needs and their current mood. This information prepares students for the appropriate tone to adopt in their facilitation approach to the session.

Engagement

We were working on our pilot digital applied theatre project at that time, and the project team felt that Jacob could benefit from taking part in the workshop. When someone is in hospital, experiencing confusion and upset, it's important to offer interventions that address the isolation a patient can experience from being located alone in a side room with little interaction. For Jacob, staff felt that diverting his attention to something creative and calming was important; this is an essential quality of the projects we offer.

The Your Story Your Way (Abraham and Ruddock, 2021: 22) project was delivered by three students on Zoom and supported in-person by the project team to enable Jacob to access the workshop calmly and with ease. The project team were aware that Jacob had a history of artistic practice; he had been a decorator and enjoyed painting and sculpture as hobbies. They integrated this information into the workshop as a "hook", to engage Jacob in a topic he enjoys. During the project delivery, there was constant communication between the project team online and the in-person team through transmedia, in order to keep checking in on Jacob's engagement and interest, and to address any issues in understanding his quieter responses. He enjoyed talking about his creative practice, and shared stories of his childhood, the forest and his love of nature. Jacob's wife also joined the workshop, and elaborated on Jacob's interests, so they were sharing ideas together as dual participants. The project team offered tasks that engaged the patient in conversations about the seasons and about colours that hold meaning, and created templates that enabled Jacob to share and structure his stories more easily.

At the end of the session, the project team on Zoom asked Jacob how he would like his story created in digital and physical forms. He was adamant that he wanted to bring the forest to life in his story. He wanted to incorporate his ideas into a poem, too, to tell the stories of his childhood through poetry – he wrote one in the session, with the support of the project team and students. The students then gathered his ideas and requests and created a video with images of forests, music from the genre he was interested in and the poem he had written as a subtitled voice-over, to show Jacob and his wife on the tablet.

Sharing back

The last part of the workshop involved Jacob being given the artefacts created by the team. The video he had been shown was presented on a DVD with printed CD cover, alongside a printed booklet that included the poem, illustrated by images of the forest. Additionally, the project team also offered bespoke craft activities to enable Jacob to make his own garden. Together, Jacob and the in-person team made a paper mache tree, fake grass, a well, birds, LED lights and model insects; it took about an hour after the main project delivery. Jacob's response to the artefacts that resulted from the project was extremely positive; he cried in delight, and called his wife to share in his response. He said that he would give his garden to his granddaughter and would never forget what the team had done for him.

After this intervention, and alongside the holistic care Jacob received from the dementia care team, he started responding more positively to the care and requests of ward staff. His wellbeing also improved, including his eating and drinking. It wasn't a huge shift, but it was a relatively significant change that may be connected to the level of empathy he received from his care with the team.

Reflect

1.   **How did the students engage the patient?**
2.   **What communication strategies did you notice in this example?**
3.   **How did reciprocity occur in this example and why was it important?**

4. **How might we read the patient's response to the students' artefact, and what does this tell us about the impact of this work?**

5. **What communication strategies did you notice in this example?**

Take some time to think about your own responses to this case study before moving on to our perspective, which may complement or contradict your own reflections. There are often many ways of seeing an event or experience, and we can always benefit from different points of view – our perspective is, in many ways, no "truer" or more valuable than yours.

Our perspective on the case study

Unpacking this scenario, we can extract several key points that illustrate person-centred approaches to practice taken by the students and the project team, which celebrate the personhood of the patient. We can see how the students used the briefing material to create connections with the patient; they found topics that the patient could relate to, to bridge the physical divide through the digital lens of Zoom. They thought about how to listen to the individual ideas of the patient in order to offer bespoke artefacts that further celebrated the artistic ideas and requests the patient had shared. They actively listened and responded to the perspective of the patient through engaging with and asking questions about the patient's interests. They also engaged with transmedia to check in with the in-person clinical team, to see if the patient was okay to continue and that he was enjoying the session. These check-ins called upon multiple readings of the patient's responses to ensure he was entering the "joy zone" of the interaction. Susan McFadden and John

McFadden (2011) recount a narrative of a geriatrician who burst into a conference room sharing her own experience of smelling the scent of her favourite flowers and remarking how this had instantly lifted her spirits. She called this her "joy zone" and explained that lists of things that make us happy – for example, sensory experiences – are vitally important to share, because they bring joy when encountered. If we know someone's favourite song or place, we can bring these images and sounds into play within digital workshops through instantaneous sharing. This approach can enable us to offer patients a sense of "peace and pleasure through the cloud of anxiety and confusion that so often accompanies dementia" (2011: 79).

Offering invitations to connect is important, and provides avenues for facilitators to meet the criteria for person-centred practices set out in Dawn Brooker and Isabelle Latham's VIPS framework.

V (Valuing people): A value base that asserts the absolute value of all human lives, regardless of age or cognitive ability.

I (Individualised care): An individualised approach, recognising uniqueness.

P (Personal perspectives): Understanding the world from the perspective of the person identified as needing support.

S (Social environment): Providing a social environment that supports psychological needs.

(Brooker and Latham 2016: 175)

Thinking about the VIPS framework and the qualities for the joy zone, take a moment to consider the following questions, to further analyse the first case study.

Reflect

1. **Can you identify each of the VIPS elements within the case study example?**
2. **How was joy apparent in the case study example?**
3. **Why is joy important for older adults in hospital?**
4. **How might joy be connected to creative practice?**

Case study #2 Stan's story
Context

[Vic] Sometimes we find ourselves in the rare position of already knowing the patients we will be working with, from having supported them or their partners before. Most of the time, though, when we ask ward staff to recommend a patient, we then meet that patient for the first time. One such patient who I remember well is Stan. Stan was in hospital for a long time. He had a love of music and travelling, he was calm and kind in his manner and he seemed very interested in sharing his stories with the project team in person and on Zoom. He was identified by ward staff as someone who would benefit from taking part in one of our projects, largely to alleviate his boredom of the ward, which can often impact how a patient feels while they are staying in hospital. Patients awaiting care home places, carer arrangements or safe navigation back home often tell us that they feel anxious and unsettled by the uncertainty of where they will find themselves next. Stan was awaiting confirmation of arrangements for his discharge from hospital, so he welcomed the distraction of an activity with students on Zoom. What the team hadn't accounted for was Stan's kindness in sharing his story, and the subsequent reciprocal generosity of several students who had returned home to a myriad of countries around the world as the pandemic hit the UK.

In the ward we were working in, there were ongoing complex challenges for ward staff to navigate, so we were unsure what reception we would get when we entered. We set up a projection screen, tablet, speakers and microphones, with our Wi-Fi hotspot and various colourful laminated resources in hand. This generated a lot of interest from patients and staff alike. We recruited two patients for our first ever pilot workshops; Stan, having been previously identified as someone who might benefit, then volunteered to be one of our first patients. He engaged thoughtfully throughout, and the project team made spontaneous adaptations to meet his access needs; for example, they used verbal description to overcome Stan's visual impairments, and scribing to capture the responses he gave to workshop tasks.

Engagement

We worked with Stan on a Medicine for the Elderly ward. It was the second workshop of our pilot project, and we were still learning how best to introduce patients to the use of tablets in wards and ensure content was accessible and appropriate. Stan took to the technology with ease, and quickly showed us how moving and inspirational his stories were. We were deeply affected by his words when he shared his memories of travelling around the world in his job as an engineer. Stan related one particular story that stayed with us; he told us that when he was younger, he wanted to travel the globe and spent time moving from country to country. On his travels he met a beautiful lady who he spent time with while he was in Italy. Thinking they'd never see each other again, he moved on with his travels, as did she, but they kept meeting in different cities on their travels every few years. This feels even more serendipitous when you remember that at the time there were no mobile phones, and neither person had a permanent address to write to. He said that over time they fell in love with one another, and he hopes that they will meet once more – this time, he tells us, he will marry her. During this interaction, the online project team noted the countries he had visited and those he still aspired to visit. They also started collating images and ideas to share back with Stan, to check they understood his location requests correctly. Stan shared his dreams of visiting many more countries on his planned future travels, but noted his concern about the possibility of such plans due to COVID limitations on travel. The team, however, had a plan to support him, and together devised an idea to bring his hopes to fruition.

Sharing back

The students, feeling emotionally moved by Stan's story, developed an idea to enable Stan to "visit" countries that he still wished to see. They called for help from classmates and acquaintances through group chats, asking everyone they contacted to create a personalised greeting from their country, especially focusing on locations where it was safe to stand in a garden or backyard or park. Stan subsequently received messages or stories from China, Mexico, Thailand, Greece and the UK – to name but a few! Each message was directly addressed to Stan, and shared the messenger's experiences of each location. The personalised nature of the videos was important; offering generic stories may not have made sense out of context for Stan, and may have simply led to confusion. When he received the video, at first Stan thought it was happening live, as the project had been, and he responded to the student messages, waving and greeting each person. Soon, though, he realised it was pre-recorded, and that he could watch again and again whenever he wanted to see it. His response was very sweet; he said that he was very happy to share his stories with the students and hoped his experience in life inspired them. He was very grateful for the film and enjoyed watching the messages, and said he'd like to keep his DVD copy to show to his sister when he returned from hospital.

Reflect

1. **How was rapport built and why was it important?**
2. **How did the group use transmedia to engage their patient?**
3. **How is person-centred care enacted in this example?**

Take some time to think about your own responses to this case study before moving on to our perspective, which may complement or contradict your own reflections. There are often many ways of seeing an event or experience, and we can always benefit from different points of view.

Our perspective on the case study

[Nicky] This example reveals how Stan engaged with the students spontaneously, to create connections that traversed the digital divide. Primarily, the connections were formed through Stan sharing an emotive story, and because the group managed to find fluidity in navigating Stan's access needs. Though Stan had a visual impairment, he felt comfortable and willing to engage with the students, to listen to their ideas and share a narrative, which was much better for him than the original plan of students showing images on the tablet screen. This naturally evolved as a strategy that Stan proposed and the students accepted as a way of engaging with oral traditions in storytelling. Even though there are structures in place in the workshop, we advise students to be flexible and follow the thread of conversation set by the patient, instead of imposing a pre-existing structure where it's inappropriate to do so. This allows the group to adapt to the individual needs of the patient – a vital component of person-centred care.

Summary of learning from Chapter 1

To summarise this chapter, we have explored the following ideas.

- The importance of active listening by thinking about the significance of being listened to and valued as an individual.
- The implications of not being heard or valued and how this is a form of malignant social psychology (MSP) have also been explored with points of reflection on how this may feel.
- We have discussed the purpose of digital applied theatre

practice, examining key features of the work and how this relates to the need for meaningful activity for people living with dementia.

- The role of the responsive facilitator and their key qualities were the subject of attention later in this chapter as a consideration of what might constitute best practice and an approach for supporting patients in residential or hospital care.
- We have found ways to offer responsive practice through the use of transmedia. We have presented an overview and detailed model to illustrate transmedia interactions that happen in digital applied theatre workshops.
- We have explored two case study examples of practice offering specific recollections of person-centred practice and responsive transmedia in action.

To complete the chapter, there is a group assignment for you to complete to upskill in transmedia communication and facilitation techniques.

Assignment suggestion: Transmedia facilitation and creative practice

Advice

- When working together to offer virtual creative practice interventions in a hospital setting, it is important to repurpose familiar technological communication tools to offer support to one another.

Task

- Split a small team into pairs.

- One person is the participant, another is providing in-person support for their engagement with a tablet/laptop/other mobile device.

- The other two team members take on the roles of creative facilitators online. (The task requires four or more people.)

- The in-person support and two facilitators need to set up a WhatsApp chat. In this chat practitioners can communicate without disrupting the session.

- The individual in the in-person support role should have a chat with their participants about their favourite places to visit and any keen interests prior to the session and then communicate these to the facilitators on WhatsApp.

- The facilitating team may wish to gather YouTube links to the location/best equivalent, photographs, sound effects or music to meet the interests of their participant. They may also create a Google Jamboard.

- The task is to create a short story and lead characters to occupy a familiar place for the participant.

NOTE: Use WhatsApp to ask questions for clarity from your in-person support, send photos to share with the participant to save multiple screen shares, prepare links to resources and note when to share them with your in-person support. Follow the ideas of your participant and use your Jamboard to document responses instantly, share images and form ideas. You may want to prepare templates for this before the session begins.

Step 1

- Start your conversation by introducing everyone on the call and offering insights about your awareness of the participants' interests. Share your gathered YouTube links, images and Jamboard as and when you intuit this to be most useful for your participants. Remember to follow the natural flow of the conversation and to think about how to link ideas to the task you have prepared.

Step 2

- Debrief your task using the following structure and ensuring everyone has time to reply

  o   What do you feel worked well in your initial use of transmedia as a team?
  o   What are the benefits of this way of working?
  o   What challenges did you face and how can you support one another to address challenges next time to adapt transmedia to work for you?
  o   What did you learn and what would you still like to know about the potential of transmedia?
  o   What advice would you give to other teams wanting to use transmedia?

Reflect

- Once you have undertaken this way of working, think about what was effective, what was challenging and how you could adapt it to make Google Jamboards and transmedia facilitation work more efficiently for your team.

2
Playful ageing (you)

The term "ageing" is often used to describe a physical change in a person over time, which is linked in the Oxford English Dictionary to "old age", "frailty" or "illness" – all words that hold negative connotations and see ageing as a process of deterioration. This perspective is perpetuated by myths around ageing in the media and through beauty industries that present the need for "anti-ageing" approaches to longer life. There is also harmful rhetoric in the news about the burden of older adults on the state care systems, which demonises ageing in society. What these perspectives do not share is the creativity of older adults in society, who are still artists, singers, actors, storytellers and fountains of experience, attributes that rightly demand respect.

Reflect

- Spend a moment putting on the shoes of your grandparents.

[Nicky] I recall my grandad telling me so many stories. One in particular that stands out to me was a tale around luck. One summer's day – I must have been around six years old – I was bored in the garden. It was too hot to cycle or play on the swings, but I did not want to go inside either. I was helping my granddad in his little glass greenhouse at the end of the driveway, gathering ripe baby tomatoes for a picnic tea in the garden later on. Suddenly, he gasped and turned to me, one hand over the other, hiding something from my sight. He was really excited, but wouldn't tell me what he had discovered. I pleaded for him to show me what he had found, and, finally, sitting on the low brick wall outside the greenhouse, he opened his hands to reveal a small stone. I stared at it, a bit confused about its significance. I asked him why he was so excited to find this stone when he had a whole driveway of gravel? He told me to look closer; examining the stone in more detail, I found a hole in the middle of the stone, which went straight through. He told me that stones with holes in, like this one, have magical properties. He said that if you collected them and protected them, you could earn a wish.

My sister was sitting on the grass making daisy chains and getting cross when she pulled too hard and they broke – again. She saw me run to the front porch excitedly to show my nan what I had in my hands. My sister, not being one to miss much, walked over to see what the fuss was about… but she just laughed at me as I told her about the magic stone. Dismissing the story, she walked off with her cup of squash. I, on the other hand, was a big believer in magic of all kinds and spent the rest of the afternoon searching the driveway for more magical stones. As I recall, I found ten in total. My granddad said we should bury them in the vegetable patch to keep them safe from magic thieves. I quite agreed, now very worried about magic thieves, and so we dug a little hole in order to plant them and keep them safe. Before we could drop the stones in the hole, however, a face began to appear in the ground. We were both understandably a bit shocked by this, so we gently continued to dig until we revealed the head and shoulders of a china doll, buried for who knows how long. This may sound a little far-fetched, but for context, my grandad lived in a little village down a lane called Pottery Lane, which had housed the local potters years before, so finding cups and plates during normal gardening activities was not uncommon. We'd never found a doll before, though! The little face looked stern, and my grandad told me it must be a guardian for buried fortunes, so we piled the lucky stones in the same spot, switching their magic for the little china doll. We never did dig up the lucky stones, and I am yet to use my wish. I'm still waiting for the time when I need it most… or perhaps I will save it to pass on to my nieces, a little piece of history and a secret buried in the vegetable patch.

This was not a pre-arranged story. No words were written; they came naturally to my granddad, who simply played along with the little game he spontaneously created, most likely to keep me busy and alleviate boredom. We devised the story together, making the legend come to life through play and magic, and the narrative has stayed with me for over 30 years. My granddad was a builder by trade, coming from generations of builders before him. He was not a writer or an actor or any other kind of professional artist, but he had an incredible imagination and took delight in creating stories. I never saw him as "old" or "frail"; to me, he was smart and funny, and I liked making up stories with him. I never felt the presence of ageing when I was with my grandad; even when he passed away in 2010, I did not see an old man in front of me. Instead, I saw my storyteller, sleeping soundly, and dreaming up new adventures for another audience. This is perhaps why I do not relate to perceptions of older adults that are linked to frailty or economic burden. To me, those viewpoints are ill-informed and reductive, and never justifiable. In fact, from my experience of older adults in my life and work, I find these views abhorrent. They dismiss the potential in older adults to make new discoveries – to be imaginative and phenomenally creative. Some people, of course, find it harder to be creative and imaginative than others, or are wary of trying something new. Yet there is often an openness in the older adult patients I have worked with to take the risk anyway just to see what happens – more so, I would say, than when I have worked with younger adults. This sense of wonder is important to embrace, and it is our duty as applied theatre practitioners to find ways to enable access to the arts. Let's see what might happen if the possibility to play is present in our exchanges with older adults.

Consider your own experience of interacting with older adults. Perhaps these are people in your family, in your community or simply everyday encounters. Think about your experience and reflect on the following questions.

Reflect

- Think about the way older adults have been depicted by society.
    1. **What do you think of the way older adults have been depicted?**
    2. **What might the impact of this perception of older adults be on society and older adult communities?**
    3. **What are your own preconceptions of ageing?**

Creative engagement can be an effective strategy to celebrate ageing. We have talked about how important creative activities are to occupy time in lonely, anxiety-inducing and monotonous hospital wards, but these activities are also a way to celebrate patient identities. The function of hospitals is to help support a person back to a level of health that means they can go home and manage, either independently or with carers, without the need for continued hospital-based treatment. However, we must not forget the importance of looking after the mind as well as the body in caring practice. Mental health and wellbeing are important for patients' recovery, as well as for supporting patients in coping with the hospital environment, where the strangeness of not being at home with familiar surroundings can be very upsetting, and where busy wards can make it difficult to feel heard.

The above is true for all hospital patients, but people living with dementia are perhaps even more at risk of confusion. It can be necessary for someone to make decisions on behalf of people living with dementia, perhaps through power of attorney, or even just for doctors and healthcare professionals to make decisions about your medical care. Almost always, these decisions are made as part of best practice in someone's care, but I know from my Nan's reflections that people talking about you and over you, without inviting you into conversations about your care, is incredibly upsetting, distressing and confusing. You can feel as if you are not really there, not really present; you might feel you have no control over your life or care, which is very upsetting. Creative playfulness offers a sense of power back to participants – even just power that's limited to a temporary interaction through a type of reciprocal exchange that invites and values ideas from participants.

Playing

When you hear the word "play", what is the very first thing to enter your mind? For many adults, the idea of play conjures thoughts of childhood, of fun and games. For some, this includes acting and the arts. Stuart Brown (2009) argues that the value of play within games and artistic experimentation is that it provides opportunities to experiment with "what if" scenarios, which can be fantastical or explorative, and without the limits of reality.

> Play can become a doorway to a new self, one much more in tune with the world. Because play is all about trying on new behaviours and thoughts, it frees us from established patterns.
>
> (2009: 92)

Brown attests that play provides possibilities to test and trial ideas, but what is especially of note here is the proposition that this process can "free" us from established patterns of everyday life. In the case of patients in acute hospital settings, this freedom is often crucial in order to help reintroduce a sense of control, or a more positive mindset. Creative interactions could potentially "free" someone from a low mood, or from the monotony of a hospital ward, by offering playful social interactions. In this way, play can be understood as the soul of social interaction for our projects, and a key priority in offering a creative, non-judgemental space in which to share stories and ideas and devise new narratives.

Incorporating play into each of our projects makes them more fun and exciting, and it can be used as a method to help us engage with our patients, specifically those living with dementia. Jill Hayes (2011) advocates for the use of creative arts with people living with dementia, noting the power and potential of creative engagement.

> Play in its broadest sense involves a creative, fun-loving attitude to life. In imaginative play we have no expectations of "rightness"; we are open to the moment and respond to it[…] It is clearly distressing to walk into a room of people locked inside the shell of their condition[…] through the creative arts we can make a strong connection touching the most closed of individuals.
>
> (Hayes and Povey 2011: 25)

As Hayes suggests, entering the realm of imagination, and offering multiple possibilities rather than "correct" answers, provides opportunities for participation without limits and without judgement. Providing projects such as this and incorporating games and play into daily activity in a ward, particularly in Medicine for the Elderly wards, has a positive impact on patient wellbeing. Our project team provide person-centered care as part of this support. We provide one-to-one or group activities, which are effective, as evidenced by the good feedback we have received not only from the patients but also from hospital staff and relatives.

[Vic] As a project co-leader, I have planned bespoke workshops for patients and then delivered these in collaboration with primary/secondary schools/students as part of our intergenerational project. Bespoke workshops offer cognitively stimulating activity for patients living with dementia, thus helping support their wellbeing during their stay in the hospital. It is heart-warming to see our patients smile, enjoy themselves and willingly participate in our projects. In this way, they feel a greater sense of belonging and feel valued. This impact is especially noticeable in, and important for, patients who are isolated. It's heartbreaking to see patients presenting a low mood, and it can make it harder for them to recover, so it is essential to be empathetic to their experience in hospital as part of our approach to developing responsive practice. One instance I recall is when a patient who was taking part in one of our workshops mentioned that he felt valued while doing so. This may seem insignificant, but what we have learnt is that impact is context-relative. In the case of this patient, he had rarely had social interactions since his wife died, and because of this he had become depressed and lost his desire to live. Previously he had stated that he frequently felt waves of sadness while living alone. This kind of story only adds urgency to the need for playful interventions that can interrupt long periods of sadness and loneliness with creativity, laughter, company and a sense of validity.

The form that play takes can be subtle. Perhaps it will emerge from imaginative "what if" scenarios, such as thinking about adventures we may like to revisit, or fantastical journeys we may go on within a fictional story as a character or ourselves. Play doesn't have to be elaborate or all-encompassing. It can simply involve listening and asking questions about an aspiration. It can be immersive in nature, or it can fall somewhere in between the subtle and the extensive.

[Nicky] I recall our Intergen project sessions taking place in a fictional village. Patients, facilitators, teachers and school children played a number of new characters online; it was the characters' job to solve mysterious events that had occurred in the imagined location. Patients would sometimes wear props or simple costumes; this could be a laminated COVID-safe detective badge, or an upside-down unused cardboard sick bowl as a hat! The inventiveness we have discovered by being limited to single-use items or items already on the ward as costume and props has enabled us to increase our creative problem-solving rather, than limited it. Here are a few examples.

- Using virtual backgrounds and screen-sharing across multiple tablets to show the patient the "case file" of the fictional village, or creating a collaborative clues board that both children and patients can populate with their theories.
- Screen-sharing computer-based audio to create a ritual. This ritual brings participants into the fictional world of the village with a simple theme song and ends the story with the same piece of music, which serves to create an immersive space in a hospital that meets COVID safety requirements.
- The use of plastic cups as telephones, or gloves full of water as chickens on a farm, works extraordinarily well to create playful worlds in a hospital. They also serve to generate a lot of laughter from the children on Zoom, the ward staff and other patients around us. We have seen many people marvel at the creativity of the patient-participants, who often suggest solutions with objects they have around them.

It is impossible to say whether this is a skill that emerges from being a grandparent entertaining their grandchildren or as a consequence of being invited to be playful and imagine a world without limits. What we can see is that playfulness, and encouraging imagination, creates a lot of much-needed joy. Creating space to enable people to play requires a level of confidence, comfort and support to allow participants and facilitators alike to take creative risks and engage in playful exchanges. It also requires a sense of equality and understanding within the facilitating team, which we refer to in our practice as a horizontal team structure.

Horizontal team structure

It is important to state that a horizontal team structure is not just needed within the facilitation team online; it is also very much part of the way we work as a whole project team to support one another. Our horizontal structure therefore includes students, clinical staff and applied theatre staff in addition to patients/residents and care home activity coordinators/supporting staff, as appropriate. The notion of a horizontal structure as a way of working is contested, particularly since it has previously been used in large-scale events – for example, in protests like the Occupy movement (see Lubin, 2012) – to assist with ideas, collaboration, problem-solving and exchanging perspectives. However, the challenges arise not in the non-hierarchical structure of this type of event but in the decision-making that is inevitably needed to make things happen. When there is not unanimous agreement within a project team, it can cause delays or conflict to emerge.

How we handle this is that in our model for a horizontal team, decisions can be made by anyone in the team. This includes decisions such as changing direction, to stay on a particular activity for longer, to add something new, to share something on-screen or to hand over to another member of the group. Our non-hierarchical structure simply means that we all agree to support the person who has made a decision and take collective responsibility to ensure that we all provide what is needed in terms of transmedia, research and co-facilitation to try out their idea. We also have a culture of learning and not blaming if an impromptu idea doesn't work in practice; when this happens, as it inevitably sometimes will, we agree to take the opportunity to be reflective and consider how we might adapt a different approach in future. We also agree that if something isn't working, then we can share this observation with the team and adapt and change tack without resentment. The idea is that we are all working with the best intention, and this is an absolute underlying assumption and agreement from the beginning of all placements.

Figure 2.1 separates out the various features of our particular approach to horizontal teamwork, which we will unpack with examples to illustrate each aspect in context.

Play

Play, as we have already discussed, is important in allowing patients to feel relaxed and supported in offering creative ideas without censorship. A horizontal structure is about taking creative risks as a collective and helping one another if someone struggles, loses their place, forgets an important element of a workshop or needs to hand over to their co-pilot (pre-decided co-facilitator) for support. For example, a group wanted to try a methodology called process drama in digital form. Process drama is a type of interactive story that follows the ideas of the participants. However, after setting up the fictional world with important context about the secret mission the participants would be undertaking, the lead facilitator forgot to mention the first clue. This facilitator became stuck; to go backwards

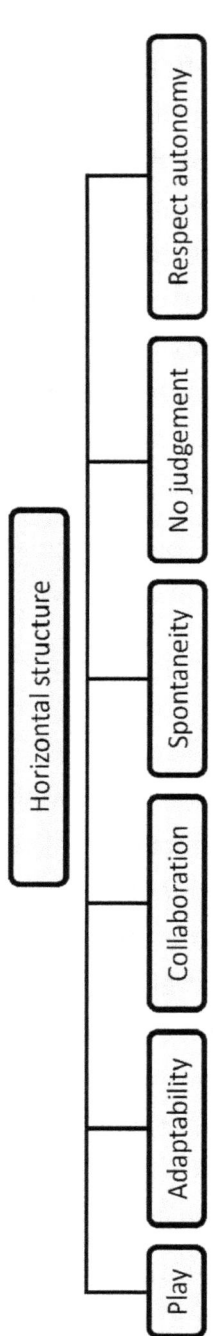

Figure 2.1 Horizontal Structure y

in the story would create confusion, but the group couldn't move forward without the first clue. Their co-pilot noticed the dilemma and improvised a solution; they stepped in as a villager in the scene, delivering the clue before handing back to the lead facilitator. In this case, the playfulness of the improvised character allowed the immersive story to continue as if it was always planned to happen that way. It also gave the lead facilitator a moment to breathe and collect their thoughts and recover from any potential flustered feelings from "messing up", while knowing that the important information had been shared. The workshop could then continue as originally planned. For that playful intervention to work, however, the group needed to collectively take responsibility for knowing the session plan inside-out. If that preparation had not been done, it would not have been a safe space for the co-pilot to take the risk. In this scenario, preparation is essential for play to take place as a support mechanism.

Adaptability and spontaneity

Play also gives permission to be mischievous and silly, for example, in responding when participants offer alternative and unexpected ways of solving a mystery that would have been impossible for the facilitation team to preconceive or predict. A horizontal structure means that we are equipped to spontaneously adapt to unexpected ideas from patients, particularly when they are interacting with children, who are also prone to offering fantastical suggestions about how a story should progress. One example took place in a workshop set in an imagined art gallery, where four pieces of art had gone missing. The patient and children collectively offered a sci-fi solution to the problem, suggesting that the items were taken by a ghost and placed in an alternative dimension. In drama, the rules of successful improvisation mean that you must not block or censor an idea, even if it takes you in a completely different direction than you had planned. Not accepting an idea can stop play from continuing, as participants feel rejected or disengaged. So, adapting in this moment, one of the facilitators took on the role of the ghost. They improvised a ritual to enable everyone to enter the alternative dimension, much to the delight of the participants, who thought this was a very funny twist to the tale and enjoyed the change of genre. Changing direction is important and needs to be allowed by horizontal team structures; we cannot hold on to a workshop plan too tightly and be responsive at the same time. The two are mutually exclusive; clinging to a plan is often a contradictory approach and can inhibit playfulness. With a horizontal team, we accept the playful reality presented and all follow the narrative – whether we are clinical staff or applied theatre practitioners – to ensure we support the creative ideas of the participants.

Improvisation is another aspect of our horizontal structure; we have seen this as a quality of spontaneously adapting practice. However, spontaneity and adaptation are not just about storytelling though; they are about being able to offer personalised and bespoke workshops that are suited to the needs of each individual patient. This means we need to avoid assumptions about how we think someone will react and be present in our practice and on transmedia to respond quickly to changes in mood, need and creative ideas. For example, recently, a patient-participant who was in her nineties and who had been a teacher for most of her life spoke to Vic before a session began about wanting to do something special for the staff on the ward. Joan wanted to thank the NHS for all they had done for her and for others in the pandemic. She shared stories of her days as a girl guide, singing to injured soldiers in underground hospitals, and said that even then she saw what the nurses were doing to support people; so she wanted to use her workshop time to develop an event to celebrate their impact. Vic briefed the students online about this, and the team began devising possible ideas, adjusting their plans and considering how they could make this a reality for Joan. However, when we arrived on the ward for the start of the session, Joan had a completely different idea in mind and had forgotten her previous suggestion; she was now much more focused on creating a video about what the students were studying instead, to allow them to share their knowledge with her. The student team, though momentarily a little worried, adapted and shared stories of their learning on their degree programme with Joan, who was delighted and offered stories of teaching in her early thirties. The group were able to spontaneously adapt by handing over to the allocated co-pilot who continued this new conversation while they adjusted their virtual backgrounds of hospitals and celebrations for the NHS, and the notes on their virtual whiteboard, instead choosing images of school classrooms and locating the schools where Joan had taught, much to her excitement. The support in the group and the continual need to adapt enabled the students to respond with flexibility and care without the need to "regroup" or to panic; instead, they intuitively followed the conversation and adapted to the chosen theme that was offered in the present rather than trying to persevere with the original topic.

Collaboration

Understanding how we might continually advance and refine our practice is important if we are to continually check in on how we are learning to adapt, respond and offer support to the patients we are working with. Once we have undertaken a project, then we engage in collective learning reflections that call upon everyone to think about what happened in the work, what worked well, what did not work and how can we adjust it for next time, what we learnt and what we need to do next. This is also a point for safeguarding check-ins, asking questions about anything that happened, observations of the ward or patients and knowledge exchange between the team to advise and support one another. What has also naturally emerged after more complex sessions where we have had to run short workshops, or if patients have experienced emotions that are more difficult to witness, for example, sadness or loss, is a genuine nurturing between the group towards one another in the debriefs. Everyone is invited to answer every question, to give their own observations and speak freely, and everyone can offer guidance, note what they learnt from each other or from unexpected moments or ask for support. We as project leads have noticed that a horizontal team structure both enables students to ask a lot of questions and offer observations and is a chance for all of us to share research and experience to guide one another through the terrain of a new digital practice. Students have also reported back to us that this way of working helps them to feel they are able to try new ideas, take responsibility, have real-world "hands-on" placement experience rather than just observing, and learn to apply theory to practice. Collaboration, in this sense, is about seeing and hearing each other before, during and after workshops have taken place.

No judgement

There are moments in workshops where things do not go to plan, despite the best of intentions. We have most definitely encountered times where students have had difficult days themselves, or struggle to explain something to a patient. For example, trying to explain VR360 to a patient in their nineties can sometimes be an easy conversation with clear examples and description; however, since virtual reality is quite a new concept, it can be difficult to explain. On our Wonder VR project, the first thing we ask students to do is to explain virtual reality films and show an example to demonstrate how it works and allow the patient to choose where to look. This often causes lots of excitement. However, with one particular patient, the students struggled to offer a clear explanation in easy-to-understand terms, which confused the patient. The students stopped talking completely, feeling worried about the patient's reactions. Vic messaged the team to take a moment to breathe, and I offered the patient a spare tablet on which to see virtual reality, which they enjoyed moving for themselves. The break in facilitation allowed the students to collect their thoughts, while I demonstrated the technology and Vic reassured everyone on transmedia not to worry. She told the team that this happens – it's complex to explain – and she invited the students to observe the patient's expression, which was one of joy. The team calmed down and continued the workshop, stating that if the patient liked the experience that I was demonstrating, they would create them one of their own to keep. The session continued without any further confusion.

In this moment, the team handed over to us as in-person support for the patient, having forgotten we had additional kit with us to help them if they wanted a live demonstration in person. This moment helped to consolidate the importance of taking a non-judgemental approach and relying on the extended team when needed, to enable access and support for the patient. The team, when reflecting on this workshop extensively, noticed their reliance on trying to hold everything themselves. They discussed the importance of not doing so when it could inhibit someone's understanding. They also expressed their gratitude that we offered support and a moment to take a step back and evaluate before they continued the session, which helped everyone to prepare themselves and not to judge themselves or one another. Instead, they were able to use the moment of pause as a learning point. This approach to learning and development helps to avoid judgement that inhibits advancing practice and experience in learning processes and forgives anything that does not go to plan instantly. After this point, we always used the in-person additional tablet to demonstrate VR to help the team, which worked well for patients and facilitators alike.

Respect autonomy

Decision-making is one of the hardest parts of teamwork, especially if you are making a decision on behalf of those you are working with. In a horizontal structure, we need to act quickly to end a session if a patient is suddenly experiencing pain or may need some other clinical intervention. Similarly, extending workshops when things are going well is also important. However, there are times when we do not know what will work in sessions, especially when we work with patients with more complex needs. For example, one patient who has a hearing impairment requested to take part in our Your Story Your Way project. We knew that the auto-transcription on the software we were using was then rather inaccurate, and so we had to adapt. We thought about other ways to get to know one another in the session and allow the patient access to the workshop she wanted to join. We asked the student team what they thought about using Google Jamboard – in particular, the post-it note function that is a feature of this software. We suggested that the team could use post-it notes to write instructions and questions, and to react to what the patient offered in return. The group were a particularly flexible team; they had excelled in previous deliveries of the project and were now quite experienced, being in their final few weeks working with us. They cautiously agreed to try, knowing that we would have to learn how to do this quickly enough to simulate the flow of conversation without being extractive or the workshop feeling like an interview.

The patient was delighted to see the students, having not seen her own grandchildren for quite some time, as visitors were still not allowed in the hospital. We used Google Jamboards as planned, but noticed quickly that too many posts were appearing, and the patient didn't know which to respond to and when. The team noticed this too and asked the lead facilitator to zoom in on the virtual post-its to help the patient focus on one at a time and to prioritise which to answer when. This worked really well. Then the patient asked for images of a particular location and pets; the team all posted at speed on the vitual whiteboard. This took some time to finesse, as it could have been overwhelming, but the patient was excited to see everyone actively listening! Once we took a second to quickly advise each other and refine this approach, she didn't struggle to understand the students. The team were very tired after the session, but motivated and excited at what they had learnt, and very pleased with the positive reaction of the patient to the communication approach they had co-created with her to suit her needs. There was no clear leader in this process, though it began being adapted by the allocated lead facilitator. Interestingly, the team were able to intuit what would work and adapted accordingly, learning from each other with every contribution. This aspect of the horizontal team structure is about respecting autonomy; by enabling the patient to contribute ideas they have autonomy to participate and respond. Similarly, the team have creative licence to adapt and try new methods of engagement – another act of autonomy. Finally, the team, working together with clinical staff and in-person facilitators, can respond openly to one another, asking questions freely without judgement in the spirit of learning and advancement and respecting one another's autonomy when working towards the same goal – in this case, inclusion.

Benefits of using a horizontal team structure

- Everyone within the team is more immediately adaptable when support is in place for all decisions and decision-makers.
- Students have reported feeling valued as equal members of the team.
- The pressure within a horizontal team structure is more

focused on developing ideas and excitement rather than risking failure, which is reframed as an essential learning process to create responsive practice.

- Students learn how to be adaptable in complex situations when a patient may have a set of ideas and access needs we need to accommodate.
- Students are more playful because they can take thoughtful risks together, knowing that they have support from everyone online and in-person should they need it.
- Students learn to collectively develop both individual and group intuition and trust.

Examples and reflection

To understand how play and playfulness are crucial elements of person-centred work, and how play can be important for older people, two case studies follow.

Read through the example case studies carefully, and then think about your responses to the reflective questions at the end of each section.

Case study #1 Adora's story
Context

[Vic] Adora was in her mid-seventies when she was admitted to a Medicine for the Elderly ward. She had undiagnosed but suspected dementia when she arrived. Her stay wasn't an easy one; she experienced challenges in adapting to the hospital environment, and because she was distressed and agitated ward staff were facing difficulties managing her care. One of the main reasons for her distress was that she missed her two pet dogs. She was concerned and worried about their whereabouts and welfare while she was in hospital; living alone, Adora's two dogs had been her only life-companions for over a decade, and she referred to them as her babies. Clearly, their company was sorely missed, and she was unsure about what had happened to them in her absence. Her anxiety grew during her stay, which caused increasing challenges for staff trying to support her. She was referred for additional support, and I was asked to work with Adora to help her to feel more comfortable in the hospital. We aimed to help her by offering a range of creative activities in addition to actively engaging with Adora about her dogs, discussing what they were like and finding out what she needed to help her feel better during her stay.

Engagement

One of the first activities I undertook with Adora was a one-to-one paper mache activity, intended to gently invite her to engage with tactile activities with me. We chose to create fake flowers to decorate her environment; this manual task also had the effect of improving fluidity of movement (dexterity) in the patient's hands. To begin this engagement, I used a conversation topic to build rapport with Adora, in this case talking about her passion for dogs, which caught Adora's attention. I also created rapport by sharing my own experience and personal stories of my own dog. Adora responded positively by engaging with me immediately, smiling, being talkative and playfully sharing her own stories about her pets. This moment revealed reciprocity between Adora and I, where much laughter ensued between us during our creative interactions. This moment also marked a turning point for Adora; she became very playful, telling jokes, sharing funny anecdotes about her dogs and creatively engaging in the activities I offered her. I noticed that the more time we spent together, the more her mood would change, and her face would lighten into a broad smile. She would beckon me to come over to her whenever she saw me, and I always obliged, sitting with her or reading with her while she enjoyed a cup of tea and a bit of chocolate. I noticed that her mood changed over time, and whenever we spent time together it was always a positive interaction. This was noticed by ward staff, who also saw a change in Adora. I always ensured Adora was happy and positive before I left the ward. Additionally, I investigated the whereabouts of her pets, and managed to coordinate with the kennels who were caring for her dogs to send photos and videos to share back with Adora. Upon seeing the videos of her beloved dogs, Adora was simultaneously happy to see her dogs being well taken care of and also tearful because she missed them. This act of kindness further established our rapport together, and I observed Adora's excitement whenever I came to see her on the ward for the remainder of her stay. Time passed very quickly whenever I spent time with Adora, and it never felt like there were enough hours in the day to hear all the stories she loved sharing with me. Chatting to me helped to calm Adora, and orientated her to the ward, including the current time, date and location, to help her recall what was happening and when.

Sharing back

This interaction led to an idea to further celebrate the connection between Adora and I to do something special and positive for her to take home from her stay. I told Nicky about my journey with Adora, and we thought about creating a bespoke song with lyrics that spoke to the process of establishing trust that had taken place during my time together with Adora. The song was titled "Have a Little Faith", and featured video footage and photographs of my time spent creating artwork with Adora. The footage also included ward staff who were part of her care and hospital journey. The photos and videos were collated and combined with footage of me singing the song to Adora, which was then presented back on the ward on a projection screen next to Adora's bed. I invited staff from the ward, including doctors, nurses, healthcare support workers and catering staff, who gathered around to watch the film with Adora. At the end of the film, the staff applauded the patient. Adora's reaction was priceless. She could not quite believe we had made this for her; she recounted a feeling of speechlessness and noted how grateful she was to have this artefact to celebrate her experience of her stay in the hospital.

Reflect

1. **How do we know that the creative activities engaged Adora?**

2. **Where is playfulness present within this example case study of practice?**

3. **Why do you think Adora's mood and interactions changed from this exchange?**

Take some time to think about your own responses to this case study before moving on to our perspective, which may complement or contradict your own reflections. There are often many ways of seeing an event or experience, and we can always benefit frcm different points of view – our perspective is, in many ways, no "truer" or more valuable than yours.

Our perspective on the case study

This interaction indicated the impact of play as a non-clinical intervention that had a clear impact on Adora's mood and wellbeing. Medicine is clearly an important part of hospital care, but play can help improve wellbeing, which may enable a patient to engage with their care and cope within the unfamiliar clinical environments in a hospital – you might call it food for the soul. Play is therefore an important offer for patients, especially those receiving palliative (end of life) care, to help people cope with potentially upsetting and frightening realities when medical solutions are exhausted. It is important to note that without building positive rapport, patients are very reluctant to engage with project team members. Therefore, building rapport is essential for effective practice working with patients. Play can, in this way, present a route to enable open conversation with patients that will support interactions between patients and the facilitators both in person and online.

Case study #2 Lorna's story
Context

[Vic] Lorna was a Filipina woman in her late fifties. She used to work as a pastor in the UK and was normally very proactive in her day-to-day life. She enjoyed going for a run in her local park and undertook housekeeping work in addition to her work as a pastor at her local church in West London. She also really enjoyed singing, particularly Christian songs with a local community church choir. She is family-oriented, nurturing close relationships with her daughter and sister through spending time together, including over Facetime during the pandemic. Lorna spent a lot of her free time enjoying *Strictly Come Dancing*, a UK dance competition with celebrities and professional dancers (known as *Dancing with the Stars* in the US). She also enjoyed watching Filipino TV, particularly soap operas, in her spare time. Unfortunately, she had a fall and broke her hip, and became disorientated afterwards, which is why she was in hospital. When I approached to her on the ward to talk about the projects she could choose to join, she showed at lot of enthusiasm for taking part in everything, despite the fact she was still experiencing pain at that point.

Engagement

Lorna chose to engage with three of our projects: Life in Lyrics, Wonder VR and Hear Me Out. During the Life in Lyrics session, she engaged with the students very well, demonstrated by her choice to sing Christmas carols and Christian songs to and with them. The students were able to use transmedia to promptly locate Lorna's favourite songs on YouTube, which she reciprocated by sharing her beautiful singing with the group. In this moment, she was smiling and enjoying the impromptu singing session with the students online. No one had been expecting the patient to sing along, but they adapted in the moment to spend time letting Lorna sing her favourite songs – in effect, performing an improvised concert for the ward. By chance, one of the students was also a singer in a similar community choir and was able to join in, much to Lorna's delight. This moment also caused staff on the ward to stop where they were and listen, sing along and complement Lorna on her great singing voice. Lorna told me how grateful she was for us taking time to engage with her, reflecting that she felt valued because the students chose to work with her.

We returned the next day to offer her more engagement, at the request of both Lorna and the clinical staff. When I came to see Lorna, she was still in pain and asked to do something to take her mind off it through engaging with our Wonder VR project. She was very excited to see the students again, and beckoned me over to her, inviting us to engage with her. The students, having already built rapport with Lorna on the first day, were now more aware of her interests and how to engage her in topics she cared about. The Wonder VR project opened avenues for conversations about favourite places to go on holiday, to which Lorna responded immediately that she wanted to go to the Philippines. The students asked where specifically, and she said the Hundred Islands. Lorna was very enthusiastic talking about her homeland, and invited the students to visit some time!

The students playfully engaged with this conversation, and used transmedia to research and share the locations she spoke about. Lorna reacted emotionally to long-lost places she missed, but enjoyed seeing the images, taking her time to survey and reflect on the locations in front of her. She expressed her love of the Philippines, telling us how beautiful it was and sharing recollections of spending time on different beaches with her family when she was little. She chose to share happy memories of visiting various attractions in the country, and the students were thrilled to hear her stories and learn more. Their enthusiasm was clearly apparent throughout the session, as conversation flowed naturally between the students on screen and the patient.

Reflect

1.   **How was play present within this case study?**
2.   **What type(s) of play did you observe?**
3.   **How did the horizontal structure work in this case?**
4.   **How might the team have further enhanced a sense of play in this workshop?**

Take some time to think about your own responses to this case study before moving on to our perspective, which may complement or contradict your own reflections. There are many ways of interpreting an event or experience; think about your own point of view before you read ours and see what you can learn from both.

Our perspective on the case study

I noticed that Lorna's mood had changed significantly by the end of the session. At the start, her mood was low, her shoulders drooped and head lowered, but when I asked her about taking part in the activity, she met my eyes with confidence, and her energy shifted. She showed excitement at engaging with us again. In the session, she was animated, calm and very open with her stories; she shared generously with the students, chatting non-stop for over 45 minutes, even though the session is usually only 20 minutes. Lorna enjoyed the session so much that the student team adapted, continued and extended the time for her to follow the flow of the conversation. We always advise students to be flexible, adapting if patients need shorter or longer interactions as requested/observed/clinically advised. Afterwards, Lorna said that she felt special that we chose to spend time with her. She told us that she was usually alone at home, so having company was a luxury that she indulged in hospital. Staff on the ward reported back that Lorna enjoyed her time with the students, which they saw translate into her interactions with clinical staff, who noted that Lorna stopped pacing the ward in pain, instead sitting down in her chair next to her bed and seeming calmer.

Summary of learning from Chapter 2

In this chapter, we have explored the following themes.

- Play and playfulness are important. Play can be subtly present in workshops with gentle imaginative storytelling and adventure creation in addition to taking place in more complex methodologies such as intergenerational process drama sessions.

- The role of play has been linked in this chapter to a sense of joy and freedom as an invitation to be creative.

- An important part of enabling a playful exchange is located in the horizontal team structure that we use to offer support to students, clinical staff and patients in their engagement with creative work.

- We create space for reflection, honesty, questions, learning and responsive practice development that presents opportunities for students to acquire vital skills in supporting one another, intuitive practice, collaboration and adaptation.

To finish this chapter, we have set you a team task using the horizontal structure in practice to apply the learning you have engaged with through case studies and reflection.

Assignment suggestion: Horizonal teamwork task

Advice

- When planning a task with a team, it's essential to think about how you will work together to ensure everyone feels heard, and that you act upon your listening to value and validate team member ideas.

Task

- Plan a short creative exercise that will encourage laughter and play as a team.
- NOTE: Try to accept all suggested ideas and see what this is like.

Step 1

- Refine your approach. Accept all ideas and act upon those that feel more relevant.

- Refine your approach again. Accept all ideas, act upon those that are most relevant and find a way of archiving those you don't immediately use, to put into practice at a later date.

Step 2

- Plan your task, identifying roles and deadlines.

Step 3

- Assign specific roles within your team to give everyone a purpose. The suggested roles are:

  o lead facilitator
  o character-in-role/co-facilitator/co-pilot
  o timekeeper
  o notetaker
  o researcher

Step 4

- Facilitate your session ensuring you listen to one another.

Step 5

- Debrief your task using the following structure and ensuring everyone has time to reply.

  o How do you feel the task went?
  o What worked well?

o   What challenges did you face and how can we support one another to address challenges next time?

o   What did you learn and what would you still like to know/how do you find this out?

o   What should you change, if anything, for next time?

o   What is your plan going forwards and how can you improve together?

o   Any safeguarding issues arising?

o   Any questions arising that you need to research?

Reflect

•   Once you have undertaken this structure, think about how it felt to work together equally. Imagine this way of working with a tutor/placement host/collaborative partner. What are the possibilities and limitations of horizontal teamwork?

3
Reciprocity and uncertainty (we)

Uncertainty in any situation can be uncomfortable. We are writing this chapter in January 2022, in a moment of great uncertainty on multiple levels. We hear narratives of the COVID-19 pandemic moving to a phase of endemic reality, which means that we are perhaps at a point in time when we need to accept and find ways to live with COVID-19 without restrictions. There is uncertainty about rising fuel prices in the UK and the implications this will have on household expenses across the country. There is also uncertainty about conflicts continuing around Brexit, and emerging international disputes. In short, the news is fairly anxiety-inducing on an almost daily basis. It is uncomfortable to be in a situation beyond our own control, where instead of having the power to overcome and dismiss it, there are no obvious immediate actions we can take to change things for the better. We can't stop international conflict, we can't convince the government to reduce tax on fuel and we can't control the pandemic.

These are huge concerns, held by a great many people. Feeling unable to make change or take action to make things "better" can feel deeply unsettling, and at times frightening. Think for a moment about what uncertainties you may face daily. Think about what it is like to sit with situations like this for a few moments. Perhaps you are already too aware of this feeling; or perhaps you have managed to avoid this feeling altogether. Now consider what you can do to feel better about the unchangeable complexities facing you. I know that my students often opt to watch a series on an online video platform, read a book or take a long walk in the fresh air. Some prefer to bake or make crafts; others like to call home and touch base with friends and family to feel grounded in situations that make them feel unsure and concerned. What are your strategies for coping with uncertainty?

Uncertainty in practice

Uncertainty is also a feature of our work on a daily basis; we rarely know which patients we will work with until an hour or so before our workshop starts. We rarely know whether they will react well to a tablet screen, even if the idea has been introduced beforehand. We don't know if anyone will suddenly feel unwell or distracted, or need any medical intervention during our time together. There are many unknowns we face each day, and these are important to sit "well" with in order to create meaningful, responsive practice… yet it is uncomfortable. Sheila Preston (2016) reiterates this point, referring to the importance of finding ways to navigate uncertainty.

> […] in the context of working in the uncertainty of dilemmatic spaces, the facilitator undoubtedly will be faced with working outside of their comfort zone of existing experience, practice and knowledge[…] No matter how one might try to control what happens, one cannot always presuppose, pre-empt, or pre-plan

what will actually occur[…] The education of facilitators might therefore consider preparing for the reality of this unpredictability and uncertainty, and the resilience required as the way forward.

(2016: 10–11)

Working in clinical environments that are often beyond our complete understanding and expertise, we need to do our best to prepare for unpredictability. We can do this by being ready to unpack what is happening in any given moment, finding avenues to offer support to each other and the patient as appropriate and practising reflection to understand why we might have found something challenging. For example, we have had many project debriefs in which student participants have felt unsettled by a patient's visible emotion in a session – such as patient participants who suddenly feel moved by something in the activity and cry in joy or sadness. Witnessing this kind of overtly emotional reaction can of course feel disconcerting, but it is the right of all our participants to express and feel however they feel without censorship. In these moments, perhaps our uncertainty stems from our cultural or personal preference for happy emotional responses such as smiling and laughter – these are emotional cues that, as a society, we are much more used to seeing. When a participant is moved to tears, however, student confidence levels in interacting with patients suddenly decrease. This is often when we do the most transmedia coaching to support our students; we want to ensure they feel calm and comforted, and are able to either continue the session or bring the session to a close as appropriate. Often, students report feeling a sense of worry or concern during and about these moments.

From our observations and conversation with students, we can see that this worry and concern come from two places – first, from empathy for the patient participant, which is a sign of a positive connection. However, they also come from discomfort at an unexpected change of tone or emotional response.

Debriefing conversations, in these moments, seek to remind students about the challenge, and the importance, of not valuing one kind of emotional response over another. It's key for facilitators to be ever ready to embrace whatever reaction the patient gives, and to offer the support needed – whether that's to change tack, to end the session calmly or to stay present with the participant until they feel more settled. All of these options are of course informed "best guesses" as to the best way to support each participant, and we may try several approaches to ensure that the participant feels positive, if they can, by the end of their interaction with us. This is where the team is so important; the different expertise of applied theatre facilitators and clinical experts can help students make decisions about the most appropriate responses.

What we have found most useful in supporting students in moments of uncertainty, alongside immediate support through transmedia and horizontal ways of working, is learning to plan responsive workshops that offer points of pause. Planning in small pauses allows for changes in direction and encourages active listening. Responsive workshops then allow students to feel calmer, because they have prepared for the possibility of changing approach to meet the needs of their participants, which are often in flux. Nicola Abraham (2019) elaborates on this point, suggesting that trusting our own reactions or intuition can help to follow participants responsively throughout a workshop.

> […] intuitively responding to the complex changing needs of each group requires practitioners to be accepting of, and able to thrive in, processes of uncertainty. This is not only located in the contexts of the participants, but also in the uncertainty that can occur in creative processes that promote participant agency.
>
> (2019: 239)

Enabling students to trust in their own ability to make responsive decisions and allow for participant agency – including choosing not to carry on with a workshop – is an essential part of reacting to uncertainty. However, reaching a point of trust where this is possible is not a simple or formulaic process. It requires confidence in moving from the beginning of a workshop to the intended outcome without following linear structures that lead simply from point A to point B. Instead, the journey from point A to point B, if we are to offer person-centred practice, is often not linear at all, and enters a multiverse of possible routes from point A to point B. To be responsive, we need to be "okay" with following the unpredictable and bespoke journeys through a workshop as they emerge.

Non-linear planning

In the previous chapter, we explored horizontal team structures as a way to enable facilitators to engage in playful interactions with one another and with their participants, as part of creative practice. Adaptability was also discussed as an important skill in following the ideas of the participant(s). Non-linear planning is another way to help prepare for uncertainty, by having in place a range of possible activities without a set structure or order. This creates a buffet of tools and exercises for facilitators to choose from, to enable them to get from the session aim to the session outcomes following the "flow" of the session. Sheila Preston (2016) draws upon the work of Mihaly Csikszentmihalyi (1997, 2013) to describe flow as "a feeling of motivation and enjoyment that comes about from the experience of being creative and challenged" (Preston, 2016: 38). In this sense, flow provides ways for us to navigate and follow the natural progression of the session by changing our topics of interest to continually engage the interest of the participants we have met. Before we do any project work on wards, Vic speaks to patients and staff to gain consent from those who say they would like to take part in workshops before our sessions begin. In these interactions, she asks patients about their interests and hobbies, and what they might like to explore in the sessions. This is a useful starting point, but we have also learnt that we shouldn't take for granted that the areas of interest revealed in early conversations will stay the same by the afternoon. Often, interests and ideas for the session have changed and developed since that initial conversation, meaning that we need to avoid being overly reliant on early details to predict exactly how the session will go. If we cling too hard to those early details in the face of new interests being expressed, the session will become stagnant and unengaging.

Before we explore the ways in which we might plan non-linear strategies, it is important to see how they differ from more conventional approaches to planning workshops in applied theatre. Please see Figure 3.1, which depicts a simple structure for a session plan.

In conventional, linear planning, we usually begin with the lead facilitator welcoming participants to the workshop before introducing themselves and their team and, when appropriate, the intentions of the session. Following this starting point, it is good practice to "check in" with participants to see how they are feeling and gauge the mood of the room before you begin a session. Often, we use a colour check-in; for example, the facilitator presents participants with an image of a rainbow and asks them to choose a colour to describe how they feel. The

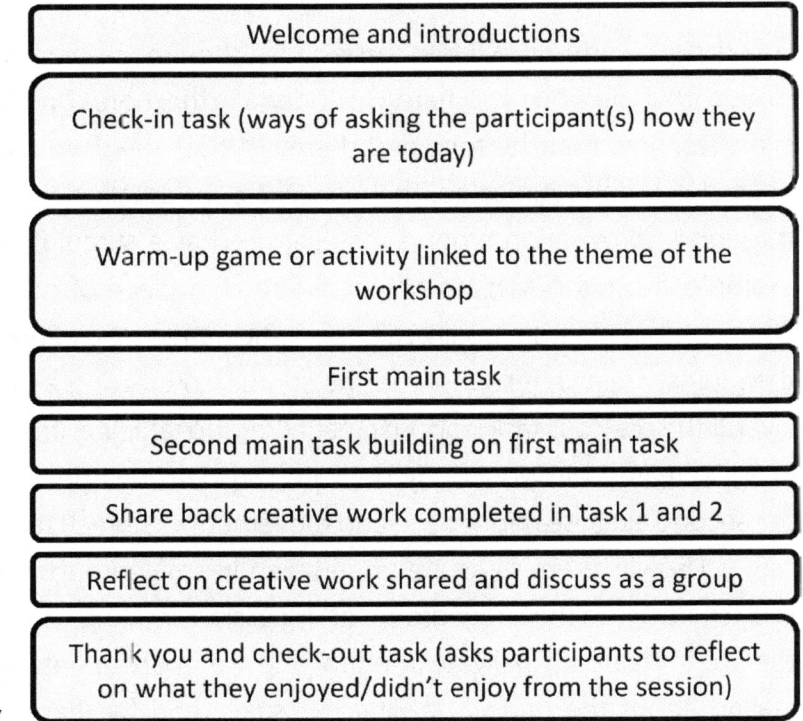

Welcome and introductions

Check-in task (ways of asking the participant(s) how they are today)

Warm-up game or activity linked to the theme of the workshop

First main task

Second main task building on first main task

Share back creative work completed in task 1 and 2

Reflect on creative work shared and discuss as a group

Thank you and check-out task (asks participants to reflect on what they enjoyed/didn't enjoy from the session)

Figure 3.1 Linear planning

key to this exercise is that you aren't necessarily reliant on the colour to communicate how the participant is feeling, but rather you pay attention to the way they say the word. For non-verbal participants, we can also read facial expressions to understand the communication of feeling in this task.

After the check-in, we usually then move into a warm-up game or activity, something connected to the theme of the session. For example, if we are going to undertake an Intergen workshop where participants explore a virtual island, we may run a collaborative seated movement warm-up, themed around tasks one might do on a ship on the voyage to the island. Maybe we mime climbing the rigging, raising the main sail or steering the ship, for instance.

Following a warm-up, a linear session plan then moves into the main part of the workshop; here, we undertake the more complex exercises, now that the tone and theme of the workshop have been clearly communicated. The main exercises usually develop through improvisation around material used as a stimulus, for example, a photograph, an object, a film or a piece of music. The second main task usually calls for participants to build upon their initial creative responses to the stimuli, so creating a new layer. If the previous task is about creating group tableaux (frozen images created with your body, depicting an idea or scene), then the second exercise might be to add movement or speech to the scene. Usually, these tasks are undertaken in small groups and then shared with the larger group for discussion and to celebrate the work created. Finally, to monitor the way participants are feeling about the project, facilitators usually end by thanking the participants for their contributions and conducting a check-out exercise, which could be the same as the check-in task as a point of comparison or could be something more evaluative to capture feedback and refine subsequent workshops.

Non-linear planning, by way of contrast, does not and cannot exist in this structure. Instead, a plethora of possibilities is often offered for participants to choose the route they'd like most to explore. Figure 3.2 offers a visual representation of this approach to planning, though please note this is a simplified diagram; often, we will create something much more detailed and extensive for our workshops. Figure 3.2 is an example of a Life in Lyrics non-linear session plan.

Non-linear planning: Introduction

The beginning of the session is similar to the linear plan, in that we introduce everyone to the patient-participant and spend time ensuring everyone understands how the session will work. Then, if we haven't ascertained how the patient is feeling, we will offer a check-in task – though it is useful to have several versions of this task ready to use, in case a colour-coded check-in is too abstract to be clear for the patient. We then have a range of tasks and activities that cater for different preferences in terms of levels of interaction and support. Some tasks will also have differentiated levels of difficulty; for example, a poetry template might start from a blank page that only includes syllable counts on each line, but we might also have templates that include sentence starters, or sentence starters with a collection of suggested words to choose from. Or perhaps a task might be based in the visual arts – a more challenging task might include a template of a blank CD cover along with drawing equipment, while a slightly easier-

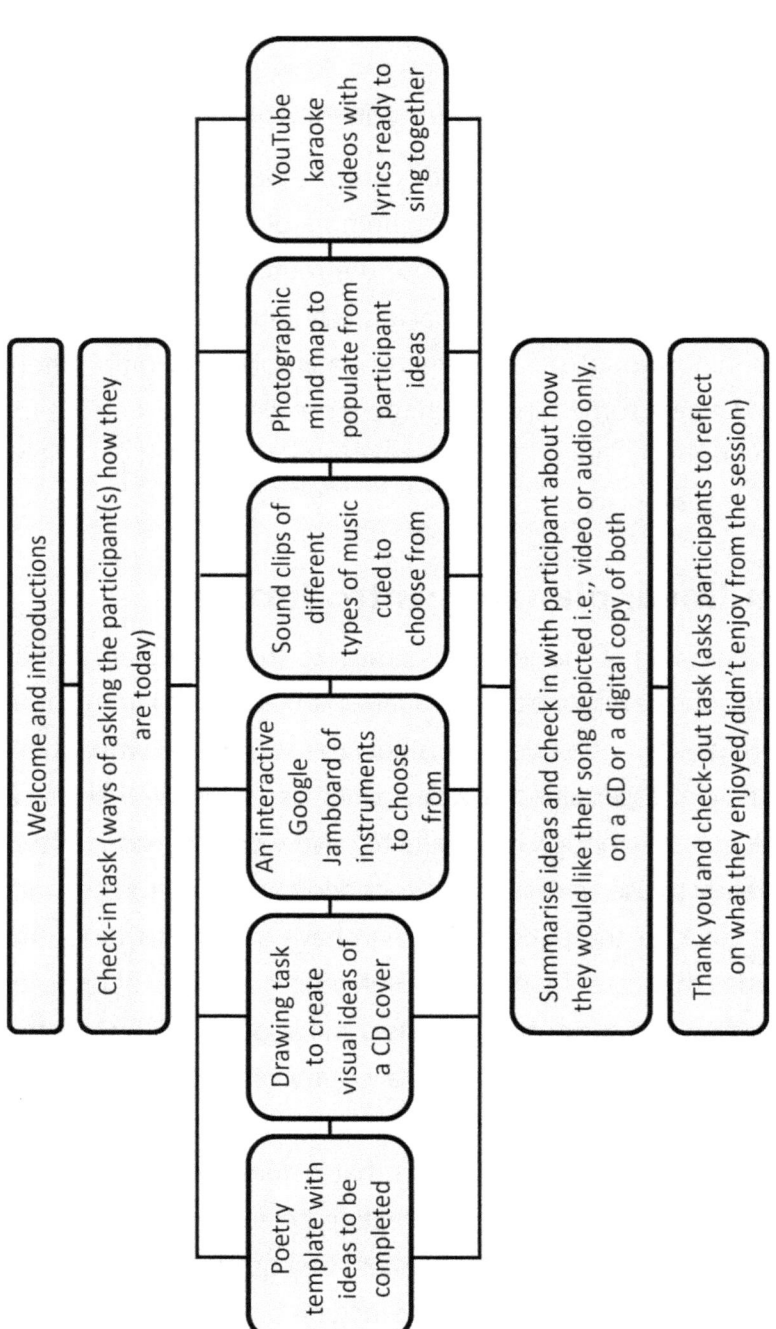

Figure 3.2 Non-linear planning

to-access task might provide the participant with glue, scissors and magazines to create a collage and a very simple version might use a digital template that allows participants to choose the colour and images they like from a pre-set collection. The examples outlined above offer a range of options for different access needs and project types to ensure the approach chosen by the practitioner is inclusive of the specific requirements for each participant. Usually, we will end up using a combination of these tasks, but we have also had sessions that are purely focused on one topic, like sharing music through singing together or creating an interactive Jamboard of ideas to form a song.

Following the flow of the session

There are also unexpected requests that we have followed when participants are excited about sharing a particular talent, skill or interest. One example that stands out to us comes from a Life in Lyrics workshop, where patient-participant Eliza chose to share her talent for identifying birdsong. The student facilitators hadn't expected this topic to arise in the session but were quick to respond to Eliza's interest and engaged her in a game of identifying birds from their calls. While one of the team led the exercise as the host of the game, the rest of the team created a shared playlist of different birdsongs and cued them up ready to play the track and reveal the answer. Eliza was very excited to play this game and had an incredible ability to differentiate different species. She enjoyed the idea so much that she asked the team to make her a game that tested her more in this area, and to incorporate a theme song based on her favourite birds. By following this idea, the team also adapted the usual resulting artefact of this workshop from the planned CD of an original song to the alternative that Eliza had requested. This example reveals the importance of actively listening, adapting and responding to patient requests to ensure the experience is bespoke and joyful for the participant. Non-linear session plans allow for and expect multiple pathways and outcomes, planning workshops this way relies on practitioners "reading" the participant accurately and following their preferred way of working. Some of this information may be possible to ascertain before the workshop by the clinical staff hosting you the other side of the screen, but it is also important to be aware that preferences change and patients may feel tired or more agitated later in the day. Being able to respond and not make assumptions, then, is a vital component of following the natural flow of the session.

Scaffolding and the zone of proximal development

Person-centred practice that responds to the different directions a workshop can take is important to offer, but, as we have seen from previous examples, this does not mean we don't make a plan. On the contrary, non-linear workshops are only possible with extensive planning. We cannot forget, then, the fundamentals of best planning practice. For example, Lev Vygotsky's theory of scaffolding is important to consider if we are to create workshop activities that support patients in accessing our various tasks. Aura Hapenciuc (2019) discusses the key elements of Lev Vygotsky's theories of education, referring to his concept of scaffolding as "the pedagogical relations between the educator and the educated, which must be created in a socio-cultural development-friendly environment, necessary to stimulate the development of the educated at the optimum level, in relation to its psycho-social resources, usable in the act of learning" (2019: 15). Hapenciuc is here suggesting that creating conditions for productive learning and engagement is very important in responsive practice. Scaffolding, we can see, means planning a layering of information to enable learners to step from one layer to the next. For example, maybe you plan a series of tasks that build up the skill level of the participant in a particular area, to prepare them for more complex tasks. For our purposes, discussing ideas or creating visual options for patients to choose from that are then used to part-populate a song template, before a backing track is chosen or a tune hummed, are ways of scaffolding the process of building a song. This approach to scaffolding follows the preference of the patient but may not be linear in nature because they follow the natural flow of the session while simultaneously building in either complexity or building towards the completion of a task, for example, writing a song.

Scaffolding in non-linear planning

Scaffolding in non-linear workshop planning takes a more meta approach. For example, we may not know the route a participant will take, but each task should be designed, no matter the order in which it is completed, to layer ideas to complete an artefact. When creating a song, it is important to understand the patient's preferred genre of music; we also need to gain ideas for lyrics from stories associated with songs. Stories should not be reliant on reminiscence, because this can put pressure on patients to remember past events, which may or may not be possible or comfortable. Instead, stories can be present associations or feelings, which can be abstract or visual and need not be word-based. The order in which tasks are completed is not important, but each task should have scaffolded layers to support the patient. This may be having an image with moveable instruments that patients can use touch-screen technologies to move to show their preferences. Discussion then could be moved to the speed of the song and the tone to give us an idea of whether or not it should have a major or minor key. The lyrics could have a template with syllable count or be random words of interest or images structured in an order to form ideas for a song. It doesn't matter the order of these tasks but each offers a scaffold to build a different part of the song to help facilitators create an artefact that the participant wants. The meta approach then is an overall view of the session with micro scaffolds built in place, some pre-determined, others improvised, to build the artefact for the session while following the flow of the session for each individual patient.

Zone of proximal development

Another area of importance we can take from Vygotsky is his approach to identifying areas of development, which are located between what a participant can and can't currently do. Lev Vygotsky defined this in-between space as the zone of proximal development, or "the distance between a child's actual development level as determined by independent problem-solving and the level of potential development as determined through problem-solving under adult guidance or in collaboration with more capable peers" (Vygotsky, 1978: 86). Alyssa R. Gonzalez-DeHass and Willems (2012) elaborates on the zone of proximal development, noting that "it is done through the social interaction between the more-skilled person and the child while they work together" (Gonzalez-DeHass and Willems, 2012: 70). Although we are not working with children but with adults, who have rich and vast skills, knowledge and life experience, the same principles of supporting learning apply. These principles are crucial to planning and creating inclusive, personalised access routes for learners – whether children or the patient-participants with whom we work. The zone of proximal development may appear in different ways that are sometimes complex to determine, so what we can do is use a "check-in" task as an introduction for the session, to determine the experience and expertise of the participant before we begin the workshops.

Here's an example. Working with Joe, we learn that he has worked in television as a film-maker for lawn-mower racing for a number of years. He tells us that he as a keen eye but isn't sure how to structure a fictional film narrative. In principle, he explains, he knows how to set up a paper edit and he has ideas for a film narrative for our Auchi Street project. Here, we have identified Joe's zone of proximal development – the gap between what he knows and what he doesn't – and we can use scaffolding tasks to help him traverse that zone. We draw upon what he does know, that is, how to structure an idea into a coherent story, and support him with storytelling exercises and strategies to draw out his creative ideas. This helps to advance Joe's knowledge of fictional narratives, builds his confidence in communicating his ideas in this way and draws upon his expertise to bring his vision to life.

Does SMART work in non-linear planning?

So, non-linear planning isn't a lack of a plan. Another thing it's not is planning without an aim or clear intention; rather, it is more concerned with offering diverse routes to that aim or intention. The goal remains the same, usually (although we must always remain adaptable), but we want to be prepared with multiple ways to get to the goal so that we can meet the individual access needs and creative vision of each individual patient-participant. Borrowing from management goal-setting strategies, conventional session planning often draws upon the SMART acronym (goals should be specific, measurable, attainable, realistic and timebound) to help practitioners and teachers alike to think through and prepare their sessions and ensure their goals, and how those goals will be reached, are clear (see Doran, 1981). Though SMART goal-setting is useful for some contexts, and is often used in schools and applied theatre workshop planning, the fixed nature of the goals is restrictive for our specific context for workshop planning that needs to be less predetermined and more open to adaptation and flexibility. Theo Winter (2015) lists the criticisms of SMART goals, noting that SMART models can be contradictory. In our case, having predetermined intentions for a workshop could mean that the patient may not like their resulting artefact because they preferred something else to the offer made in the session. Similarly, it doesn't account for uncertainty, which is part of this context. Not achieving a goal can, as Winter suggests, decrease confidence in those attempting to equate success with fulfilled goals. Whereas, in our work, success is the patient feeling happy and engaged in cognitively stimulating tasks, it is not the completion of specific goals that will enable this to happen.

In our experience, it is more likely that the responsive approach that adapts, redefines intentions and actively responds to patient ideas and interests creates the most joyous experiences. Further to this, for new practitioners learning how to work in contexts that can be uncertain, Zofia Niemtus (2018) draws upon Rachel Lofthouse, suggesting that the model of SMART goals can place responsibility on an individual to affect change as if this was a straightforward "one-to-one transaction". We see this in the hospital and in care homes too, where care is multifactorial and how someone feels may be partly a response to a workshop but is often more holistically informed by the rest of their day, how they are feeling, if they are in pain, if they are missing people and so on. SMART goals, though intended to help organise and set targets that are clearly useful in many contexts, are not responsive or holistic enough to suit our specific purposes for responsive practice in this particular setting.

Why doesn't SMART work for hospital contexts?

If we break down why each element of SMART is not useful for the nuance of responsive practice in hospitals, it is important to address each point in turn. If we were specific, we would potentially shut down creativity because we wouldn't easily be able to follow the often-evolving interests of our participants; similarly, if we can't be specific, we can't be measurable, because we don't know what the outcome of the session will be. However, we may be able to see if the participant enjoyed the session as a measure of impact rather than a specific learning outcome, which isn't the focus of our approach to working. Attainable is another complex theme. We need to ensure what we devise as an idea with our participants is possible, but we also know that some patients will vary in how much they would like to communicate ideas with us despite adaptations to access needs. In this case, we need to be thinking more along the lines of how we can best meet the artistic requests/vision of the patient to make sure the project achieves what we discussed with each individual. Realistic is a good goal, and one we need to keep to, though we can't plan for it in the same way we would a session in a school, where predictions of what will happen in a class, what will likely be discussed and contributed, are possible. Timebound is the final element of the acronym and again one we can't be fixed to because though our sessions generally aim to be 20 minutes in length, in reality we may also need to extend or shorten these for each individual depending on how they are getting along, if they are in pain or if they are enjoying the conversation and would like more time.

Replacing SMART with FAIR

Replacing SMART, we use FAIR as an acronym to explain our approach. Fair stands for flexible, achievable, intuitive and responsive. Flexibility is at the heart of workshop design for non-linear planning because it presents a means of adapting and being open to the uncertainty adapting to patient ideas "in the moment" can bring. It can be calming to think flexibly about practice in clinical contexts to prepare for unknowns or sudden changes in patient needs. This can ensure everyone is equipped with the skills needed to change direction and follow the natural flow of the session. Similarly, what is achievable will vary for each patient. It is important not to make promises to patients as artists that cannot be kept. For example, promising to make a full feature-length film for a patient may not be a realistic goal, but a trailer of two to three minutes about the proposed film idea is achievable. Achievable as a feature of the FAIR acronym isn't only about what you can achieve as an outcome of a workshop but also about ensuring you are thinking responsively about the access needs of the patient and how to enable them to achieve what they'd like to within the limits of the session. A way to navigate this is through intuition and trusting yourself and one another to read and respond to clinical advice you are given through transmedia communication and also through watching for changes in expression that may signal tiredness, pain, excitement or engagement for your participant. Intuiting where to follow a thread of conversation that suits the interests of the patient is just as important as knowing when a thread has come to an end and a new topic is needed to maintain engagement. This helps to create a responsive approach to practice that puts the participant at the heart of the work.

Pedagogy of reciprocity

Another important element of our practice is located within our pedagogy of reciprocity (see Abraham, 2021b). This is based on a conceptual framework combining reflexivity, a relational ethic of care, person-centred care, co-intentionality and play to form a way of working that encourages exchanges of ideas and care in creative practice. Reciprocity may be seen as an exchange of sorts, and concerns the way that we share ideas, memories and creative suggestions and solve problems together rather than placing all the emphasis for offering any of the above on our patient. If you are not used to creative engagement, then it can seem a rather daunting task so what we need to think about as practitioners is a way to supportively encourage and take this risk ourselves. By "risk" I don't mean sharing a deeply personal story or account, but rather "modelling" or demonstrating, an idea to help support our participant to understand the intention or direction of a creative exercise. For example, if we are devising a narrative for Auchi Street, it may feel overwhelming to ask the participant to simply provide a new story from scratch. Instead, we may begin with a discussion about our favourite narratives, whether in films, books, radio dramas, podcasts, TV series or any number of other storytelling media. Reciprocity is embedded into our practice by sharing first, for example, offering a story we cherish as practitioners and sharing this with our patient. We may then ask their opinions about the story, if they know it, or, if not, what they think about the description we shared. Should the patient like the narrative, we may then follow up by asking if they know similar stories or if they like the genre of the story. If the patient doesn't like this narrative, they may be asked if they prefer another genre, with options available visually to help support patients with their choice. This element of reciprocity invites co-intentional sharing where participant and practitioner learn more *about* one another *from* one another.

Another element of reciprocity is play. We need to be playful if we are asking our patient to engage in play; otherwise, what is the fun of the exchange if only one person is playing, without reciprocity? If we are engaging in play, this can take many forms, as we have explored in previous chapters. For example, play doesn't have to be noisy and energetic; it can be calm and curious. We may, for example, be playful in the way we use virtual backgrounds, filters and augmented-reality features of the virtual video platform we are using to engage with our patient. When building characters, we can give the patient creative control to set the scene by choosing a setting that can become a virtual background in minutes. Similarly, directing the gestures, mannerisms, posture, voice and personality of characters can be playful, with one allocated actor in the call performing the ideas of the patient, which they can review and shape in real time. We can also add filters with elements of augmented-reality costume and/or make-up to add further detailed and playful engagement to our character-building experience. Saying "yes" to ideas from patients as a simple tool of improvisation provides opportunities to enhance engagement and illustrate reciprocity through active listening translated into instant visual responses through the development of characters.

A relational approach to person-centred care acknowledges the importance of making experiences bespoke to the needs of each participant. This approach also means that understanding access and inclusion is central to reciprocal practice to enable participants to engage in creative exchange. Reciprocity in this sense means finding a way to support a patient to engage, acknowledging that this is a collaborative experience of support to enable freedom of expression. Take, for example, a patient with a hearing impairment who would like to engage with our digital project Your Story Your Way. In this project, the patient has autonomy over their story development and the representation of their story in the form of their choosing. However, the subtitles on the platform aren't always accurate and often appear in small text that is difficult to read. This means we need to find another way to practice that doesn't rely on spoken exchange but offers the same level of cognitive stimulation for the patient. For example, using additional tools of communication like virtual whiteboards to communicate questions in large text and sharing back responses with emojis and clear gestures of support or agreement, for example, nodding or putting a thumb up, when working on online video platforms can be an effective strategy to support the patient. The patient can then choose how they would like to respond, which may be vocally or through writing on a physical whiteboard or making choices by pointing at images or text-based choices on their screen. The patient's choices can then be communicated back to the online team by the facilitators supporting the patient in person in hospital.

A reflexive approach is required for practitioners to reflect upon their learning and to share back what they appreciated from their time with the patient. Often, we end our workshops with a circle of gratitude, with each practitioner offering a thoughtful reflection on an idea or suggestion they learnt from the patient. The patient is invited to respond and asked if they would like to share any thoughts too. This element of reflexivity asks practitioners to think about their experience and offer meaningful reflections with their participant. Another element of reflexivity must come after the session to ask practitioners to think critically about their workshop approach: whether it worked, what they might change, what they learnt – there is always something new to learn – and how they are feeling. This type of debrief requires practitioners to think about their own cultural beliefs and politics, and how these may or may not have played out in workshops where they may have felt uncertain about something that was said or something that happened in the fictional world. It is important to unpack these moments, which can sit with practitioners and cause problems or hesitation, lower confidence or impact choices in future workshops. Deep reflection can help teams to be honest and supportive of one another and invite questions for clinical partners who will have a different and more complex perspective on interactions from a medical perspective that can help practitioners understand how to improve, feel calmer or change practice in future.

A reciprocal approach is not advocated as a strategy to expect responses or offers of ideas from patients, but often patients are more receptive to sharing ideas with the team if they feel we are sharing too and are prepared to take that risk first in proposing a story to share. This can be as simple as "modelling" or "showing" an example to illustrate a task. For instance, if we are asking participants about their favourite holidays, we usually start by offering our own, stating, for example, that a family holiday to Cornwall to see my Nan and explore a treasure hunt for foo's gold in the Cornish Goldsmiths used to be the highlight of my summer, alongside walks on the beach and digging in the sand. We would offer this type of story to additionally provide ideas to help support participants to connect with us if they felt similarly or held similar preferences for a seaside holiday. This also helps ensure the practice isn't feeling like an interview that takes ideas, which we call an extractive model of practice, without giving anything in exchange from the facilitation team. Building trust over Zoom on tablets isn't a simple process and requires us to find ways to offer points of familiarity to build positive creative rapport with patients. Finding ways to do this through responsive practice as a way of acknowledging and responding to ideas is essential to ensure we are acting in opposition to harmful and patronising rhetoric about dementia.

> It is vital that the pedagogical approach we take is in itself a political act that provides a positive counter narrative of people living with dementia as artists who are greatly valued and actively listened to in relational practice that challenges ageism by disrupting expectations of what is thought to be possible through creative engagement.
>
> (Abraham, 2022b)

Reciprocity is then an opportunity to action the above intention through sharing and being open to following the interests of the people we are working with. Reciprocity can be located both in our creative offers to share stories and in our adaptable way of working through non-linear practice.

Examples and reflection

To understand how transmedia and a person-centred approach work to celebrate personhood in practice, two case studies follow.

Read through the case studies carefully, and then think about your responses to the reflective questions at the end of each section.

Case study #1 Margaret's story
Context

[Vic] Margaret was admitted to hospital after a nasty fall left her in pain. She was experiencing low moods during her stay due to the ongoing pain of her injury despite being given painkillers. Margaret was referred to me by nursing staff, in the hope that I could offer a diversion from her pain through non-medical interventions. Distraction from pain is very important for recovery; increased pain can cause agitation and less engagement with staff, which can also result in the rejection of food and drink and a lack of sleep. All these factors can manifest in delirium, which is an acute form of confusion that is disorientating for patients and often increases hospital stays and recovery time. When I first met Margaret and asked her if she would like to join the workshops, she initially declined, saying she was in too much pain to do anything, and asked me to come back another day. She also expressed that she was upset because she was missing her sister, who she usually saw frequently. I returned to Margaret, as promised, since the staff re-referred the patient for support. That day she had a visitor, her sister, who improved her mood significantly. When I saw her sister was about to leave, I asked once again if she felt up to joining our workshops that afternoon; this time she happily agreed to take part. To understand Margaret's interests, I spent time with her, asking about her interests, to enable the project team to tailor the afternoon workshops to her needs. Margaret related to me that she really liked the arts, specifically dance, having been a dancer for a local company in her youth. She also shared with me that she was a nurse in a London healthcare trust for the army, looking after injured soldiers who had returned from warzones around the world, before changing career later in life to work as a personal assistant in a local business. I related this information back to the student team via transmedia to inform their topics of choice ready for the afternoon workshop.

Engagement

In the session, I returned to see Margaret and checked in again that she was happy to join our workshop. She was sat up on her bed smiling at me as I walked towards her, commenting that she had been waiting for us. I responded, saying that was great and we were excited to work with her. I introduced the students to Margaret, and the students took over, facilitating and talking her through the project. Margaret was engaged immediately because they used the information I had given to them prior to the session; straight away, the students were able to talk about topics that she had previously expressed interest in. Because of this reciprocal sharing, the session went really well. During the workshop, the conversation flowed naturally between the facilitation team online and Margaret. Margaret really enjoyed sharing her life experiences with the students, and the students were in awe at her achievements and the moving stories she shared about her time as a nurse caring for injured soldiers. Usually, at the end of the session, students ask their patient how they would like their stories represented as an artefact for the Your Story Your Way project. Unusually this time, Margaret requested a different outcome from this session; she asked the students to make something about themselves, so she could learn more about their stories and their experiences of the arts.

Sharing back

The students were a little daunted by this unusual request, but, having spoken to Margaret about her hobbies, they proposed that they could create a podcast for her like the radio shows she enjoyed listening to as a way to share their stories with her. Margaret liked the sound of this idea, so the students worked together to share short three- to four-minute narratives about something that they were most proud of, and a short story about how they had been inspired to study applied theatre at master's level. This was constructed as a question-and-answer session with a host to guide Margaret through their stories. Margaret was discharged from hospital shortly after our workshop, so the group wrote a letter recapping our time together in the workshop and created a CD for her to listen to the artefact they had created for her.

Reflect

1. **Where did reciprocity take place in this case study?**
2. **How might the team have increased reciprocity in their final artefact?**
3. **How did the team use the non-linear planning of their session to adapt to the needs of the patient?**
4. **What might the FAIR objectives be for this session?**

Take some time to think about your own responses to this case study before moving on to our perspective, which may complement or contradict your own reflections. There are often many ways of seeing an event or experience, and we can always benefit from different points of view – our perspective is, in many ways, no "truer" or more valuable than yours.

Our perspective on the case study

From this example, we learnt that reciprocity can take many forms. On one level, reciprocity happened before the workshop began, with the initial transmedia sharing of stories that were then integrated in the start of the project. This moment demonstrates a clear investment and interest in Margaret's story by the student team, who had prepared questions, images and ideas to share with her to help everyone connect from the start of their session. Reciprocity also occurred when the patient offered more stories to the team, and when the students suggested ideas to put the patient's request into an action plan. Instead of panicking at the unusual requests, the team instantaneously switched their approach and accepted the offer of an idea for the patient, and reciprocated her stories with their own.

Case study #2 Dev's story
Context

[Vic] One of our frequent project locations is an acute dialysis ward, where patients have various cognitive impairments. There, we usually deliver our collaborative film project, Auchi Street. Patients undertake dialysis three times a week, and though this is essential care it can also be disruptive for patients' sleeping patterns. It is a tiring process, and often means that people sleep in the day rather than at night. Similarly, this is clearly disruptive to everyday routines, and can impact the wellbeing of patients undergoing this treatment. Supporting patients while they are undergoing dialysis, with activities that can keep them awake and creatively engaged, is a way of improving patient wellbeing while they are undergoing this treatment.

The ward we usually work with had a very challenging week in the autumn of 2021. In one particular week, the ward experienced several patients dying, causing much grief for the staff and fellow patients, who had known each other for a lengthy period of time. The impact of this, in the second wave of COVID-19 in the UK, had taken its toll; frustrations and tensions were increased and were impacting the wellbeing of many in the ward, despite incredible efforts from clinical staff to support everyone. At this point, we were reaching the end of our collaborative film-making process, where the one-to-one work done with patients is then fused together to form one super-narrative celebrating multiple ideas across several dialysis sessions.

Engagement

In one of our last sessions, we were showing the patients a trailer for the film we had been working on together. We were excited that in this version, a patient had also performed in the film as the character he had created. However, upon seeing the trailer, one of the patients, Dev, told us that he was not happy that this person was in the film; further information revealed a historical feud between him and our actor, based on past disagreements. The team were in the middle of the session at this point, at the end of the project, and were unsettled by this unexpected information. The sudden change of reaction – from a previously positive experience, with patients being unanimously excited, to a conflict – was off-putting, and worried the team. They were concerned about the impact of this unexpected moment on the future of the project and, most importantly, on the wellbeing of this patient.

In discussing the trailer, the patients had been made aware that they could request changes to the film at any time, so there was an opportunity for a conversation about how to resolve this matter. The team needed a resolution that meant everyone still felt part of the film and also had their concerns taken seriously. The patient who raised this issue responded well to the conversation and was happy to suggest ideas to address this for his version of the film. This meant that Dev was happy to continue working on the project, knowing his changes would be enacted.

Sharing back

For the film premiere, we made an individual version of the final film just for Dev; in his version, another actor played the contested role. The other copies of the film held the original recording for the patient who performed his character's part. When he watched the film back, Dev was tearful and grateful for the final version of the film, with much excitement to see his character and scene woven throughout the narrative of the film. He told us that he was really happy with the final outcome of the film and accepted his copy of the script, trophy and certificate with tears of happiness. This "goodie bag" – containing the final version of the film, a transcript of the film, a certificate of participation and an accompanying trophy – is an important part of the project. Sharing artefacts that document the filming process, to commemorate the ideas shared in the process of creating the film, is an important step in ensuring that patients are located centrally as artists within the project from start to finish.

Reflect

1. **Where was uncertainty located within this workshop?**
2. **How else might you respond to this situation in a way that shows active listening?**
3. **What was the impact of the team adapting to the requests of the patient?**
4. **How was FAIR present within this moment of practice?**

Take some time to think about your own responses to this case study before moving on to our perspective, which may complement or contradict your own reflections. There are often many ways of seeing an event or experience, and we can always benefit from different points of view.

Our perspective on the case study

We have a no-exclusion policy in our practice, inviting all patients to take part if they choose to do so. It is important that this offer to participate is extended to as many patients as possible to keep people awake, cognitively stimulated and creatively engaged in something exciting that celebrates different ideas. We were unaware of the difference of opinion that had elapsed in the past between two of the participants because changes had already been made to ensure both patients were comfortable in different dialysis time slots. Emotions were also heightened at this point in time due to the deaths on the ward, but the situation was easily resolved with a conversation to create an alternative approach to representation in the collaborative film that satisfied both patients. The patient who was unhappy with the casting still liked all the shared ideas and narratives developed by their co-collaborators. Listening to his concerns, we were able to ensure he felt heard and was enabled to suggest his own version of the film. This was a strategy to solve the conflict that worked well in this example, ensuring both patients were happy and involved in the way they preferred for their individual representations of the collective narrative they developed. This simple gesture helped to support the patients through not only listening to the issue one of them identified but also taking this seriously and offering a conversation about how he felt the issue could best be addressed to resolve the challenge he had brought to our attention. Disagreements can happen from time to time and it's important to maintain a safe space to discuss what can be put in place to support everyone should this occur; this will necessarily be bespoke to each circumstance.

Summary of learning from Chapter 3

In this chapter, we have considered the following.

- Insights into non-linear planning which offer a comparison with more traditional linear versions of session planning workshops.
- It is important to acknowledge and understand how uncertainty is present in our lives and practice and that this can feel uncomfortable.
- It is important to have strategies in place to think about how to embrace and follow the flow of uncertainty when we are working in different contexts.

- Embracing uncertainty will help us to become active and responsive practitioners who are ready to adapt to put the needs and ideas of our participants at the forefront of our practice.

- We have also discussed the theme of reciprocity and how this can be present within both our creative exchanges with participants and also within the offer of flexibility in our practice.

The tasks we have included in this chapter will ask you to think about your own practice and how you can embody a reciprocal approach to creative work through following the thread of an idea to fruition.

Assignment suggestion: Reciprocity and improvisation

Advice

- It is important to think about how to provide points of connection between participants and practitioners co-inhabiting virtual spaces through reciprocity. This is essential to avoid extractive practice that takes ideas without offering a sharing space for patients.

Task

- Working in pairs, label yourselves A and B. Next, write down a number of questions you want to ask each other. Here are some examples to help you, based around a song you both know.

  1   What is your favourite genre of music and why?

2   Where did you first hear this song?
3   How does this song make you feel when you hear it?
4   Does this song bring any stories to mind?
5   Can you tell me about the stories it provokes for you?

Step 1

- In this task, person A will ask the questions and person B will respond.

Step 2

- Person B will then ask their set of questions, but this time A and B will share their answers. In this second scenario, if natural connections emerge, follow the conversation and see where it takes you.

Step 3

- Debrief your task using the following structure and ensuring everyone has time to reply.

  o   What was it like when you were the only person answering questions?
  o   What was it like when you both responded to the questions?
  o   Did you find any connections between your answers/ experiences?

Reflect

- Once you have undertaken this way of working, think about what was effective, what was challenging and how you could adopt a reciprocal approach in other tasks you may want to undertake with your participant group.

Assignment suggestion: Responding to uncertainty

Task

- In a team of four, working in pairs, two people will take on the role of lead facilitator and co-facilitator and will run a story-writing task for their participant. The other two members of the team will take on the role of the patient and a member of clinical staff.

Step 1

- Allocate the role of facilitator, co-facilitator, patient and clinical staff member to the members of your team. The facilitator and co-facilitator should prepare the following.

    o   Design a five-minute storytelling exercise; try a game that is carefully scaffolded and involves a gentle introduction to building a narrative that is word-based.

    o   Plan several different versions of the task using images, key words and material that can be printed and given to the member of clinical staff working with the patient.

    o   Make sure you model the task and demonstrate the ways the patient can choose to interact with the screen and/ or any other resources you have prepared for the task

    o   Try to use the digital tools on the platform you are using to make the task playful and engaging with the patient to ensure the exercise is cognitively stimulating.

Step 2

- Set up your Zoom screen with the facilitator and co-facilitator online in one room, and the patient and facilitator in another room with a laptop or tablet on a table in front of them.

Step 3

- Run the task, but for the person playing the role of the clinical staff member, at some point in the workshop choose from the following interruptions to the session and plan a response from the patient.

  1. A healthcare support worker needs to conduct observations, for example, take the patient's temperature and blood pressure.

     o Patient response option 1: The patient is annoyed by the interruption and asks the facilitator and co-facilitator to come back in ten minutes.

     o Patient response option 2: The patient is happy for the observations to happen while they stay on-screen.

     o Patient response option 3: The patient asks to stop the session and says goodbye to the team.

  2. An alarm goes off in the ward; the healthcare support worker seems concerned and is seen by the online team to be looking around the ward.

     o Patient response option 1: The patient is distressed by the noise and is struggling to hear the group.

     o Patient response option 2: The patient is indifferent to the sound and doesn't seem to be aware.

  3. The patient suddenly complains of pain and needs medication.

o   Healthcare support worker option 1: The healthcare support worker asks the group to end the session immediately.

o   Healthcare support worker option 2: The healthcare support worker messages the team that the patient will need to take medication and rest so they have five minutes to end the session.

4.   The patient is in the middle of sharing a funny story but struggles for a word, and then feels upset.

5.   Use one or a combination of scenarios to help one another practice responding thoughtfully, calmly and supportively to the patient and healthcare support worker. Use transmedia to communicate and ask questions as needed.

Reflect

•   After the task, reflect as a team about how it feels to respond to unexpected scenarios and think carefully about what worked, what didn't work, what you learnt and how you can advise one another with strategies to support everyone and feel calm in similar situations.

Conclusion

Throughout this book, we have shared insights into our evolving digital applied theatre practice and projects, offering case studies of the core ideas we have presented. We have detailed a range of topics that are important to us and our practice, having emerged from the need to adapt, be spontaneous and follow person-centred principles of practice. Our exploration of working digitally in applied theatre has taken us on a journey to explore the meaning of play for digital applied theatre practice and practitioners, focusing on not only how we might understand play but also about how we can use horizontal team structures to enable play to happen online. These topics have enabled us to deliver digital applied theatre practice in a pandemic across acute hospitals and supported living contexts. The learning we have shared with you offers real experiences of practice, learning, challenges, adaptations and interactions that we hope provide helpful insights into adapting practice to be responsive, COVID-safe and vital in supporting the wellbeing of older adults living with dementia.

An important part of this process has involved having a supportive team dynamic and non-judgemental approach to learning that have been essential components of our process to develop and advance our work. Without a supportive team, we could not have discovered the learning we have been fortunate to experience. The horizontal team structures we have developed were not pre-planned when we began the process of adapting in-person practice into digital online projects. Instead, the horizontal team structure we have shared with you evolved thanks to the consistent feedback of the student teams who took part in our projects and the project team who supported the delivery of practice to patients on wards in the pandemic. The need for a horizontal team structure comes from a position of care and compassion for our fellow practitioners in what has been an incredibly challenging few years. The learning from this time will not mean, however, that as soon as we can move back to in-person practice, we will do so; in fact, we have learnt that digital versions of our project mean we can react faster to patients and patients have reported to us that they prefer online interactions because they are less invasive and the creative potential of the media we use has meant that we are able to creatively respond to ideas dynamically with instant results. The engagement of patients with digital projects has been very positive, leading us to develop increasing models of practice to offer reciprocal exchange between generations online.

The theme of reciprocity is another layer of learning we have developed to evolve a responsive pedagogy that allows us to share safely with our participants to build rapport – even if we are physically distanced – via Zoom. We have learnt to communicate without interrupting the session for the patients we have been working with through the integration of transmedia in our practice. Transmedia hasn't only offered us a way to ask questions and give support, but allows us to cue screen-sharing, disseminate links to Jamboards and YouTube videos and share research to help support practitioners leading sessions. It has offered a route towards supportive and active teamwork for practitioners working online and is informed by clinical knowledge to help us navigate hospital wards with care, compassion and safety at the forefront of our practice. There are many important take-aways from our experience that we have shared throughout this book, and we hope you find them useful as you research or develop your own ways of navigating online practice. In this final chapter we will summarise the key elements of the fundamentals of the practice we have developed.

The fundamentals: Key points

When working in partnership with healthcare providers, you must always follow and adapt your practice to clinical guidance. Working with a clinical member of staff with knowledge of the clinical or care settings is essential. It's important to remember the following.

- **Clinical staff know the environment.** Clinical staff are well versed in navigating wards and other clinical staff and in seeking consent from patients. This is not a process you can undertake without a clinical member of staff, so it is essential to engage with healthcare staff and build this into your way of working together.
- **Clinical staff can guide you through best practice, support you and help you to follow hospital guidance.** Hospitals and care homes are complex contexts with rules and regulations to keep everyone safe and well. Clinical staff can field your questions and help you develop your practice. It's important that they are involved in your planning, implementation and debriefs to help you to evolve your practice to suit the needs of healthcare contexts, and most

importantly the patients or care home residents you are working with.

- **Work with your healthcare partner to risk-assess your activities, equipment and any other factors they identify.** This is important for any applied theatre project. You must have a robust risk assessment in place prior to the start of any project. This can be updated as you develop your work and want to try new ideas, but keep checking and rewriting it before you do any new activities with your partnership to ensure that what you would like to do is safe for your participants and your team.

Find ways to work safely and supportively with your team

Working online isn't everyone's first choice, but we have found that, actually, it's our favourite choice! It is less intrusive, less disruptive than in-person practice on wards and more engaging for patients. However, finding ways to manage this type of practice is really important to ensure you feel supported and always support one another. It's important to think about the following.

- **Find ways of communicating together without interrupting a session.** We have found that the use of transmedia is effective to support students and enable them to ask questions while maintaining responsive practice on Zoom.
- **Test your tech.** One of the most stressful parts of online working is often when your technology doesn't behave as you expect. To counter this, we ensure everyone has links to media to be shared, that those with the strongest Wi-Fi

are ready to screen-share and that there are back-up screen-sharers ready should anyone's internet stop working. We also have resources printed in case screen-sharing isn't possible. We ask the group to log on to the platform before we start sessions to practise sharing sound, video and images too. All of these measures are simple and quickly become part of our team culture. They also help reduce stress for the team.

- **Take regular breaks.** Facilitating online can be tiring. We often communicate access needs and interests of patients to students on WhatsApp prior to a session and use voice notes for questions and answers to avoid unnecessary additional screen time for the team. After the session, we also take a break away from the screen for everyone to rest and get a drink or snack so that they have time away from the session to reflect and collect their thoughts.

Person-centred practice

Person-centred practice is important to build into your projects. This will help you to design a project that locates the needs, interests and ideas of your participants at the heart of your work.

- **Person-centred practice values the person you are working with.** This is very important as a way of working that values and locates the person you are working with at the heart of your practice. Make sure you are well versed in what person-centred practice means. We have offered some insights into the need for person-centred practice in dementia care but research is always changing and advancing, so keeping up to date with the latest guidance is therefore a must. When you have created your project and session plans, make sure you talk to your clinical partnership to ask for their feedback and guidance to ensure you are on the right lines.

- **Active listening is an important part of person-centred care.** Make sure you are actively listening and think about the best way to show this through the creative practice you are offering. Consider using visual tools like Jamboards, or interactive whiteboard functions built into the platforms you are working on or that are available online to support the way you build creative ideas with your patients. Give feedback, summarise what you have been talking about and ask questions to show that you are listening, interested and thinking about how best to develop the ideas that have been shared with you.

Inclusive communication is vital to ensure you are meeting the access needs of your patients

Asking clinical staff for guidance on best communication techniques, completing online dementia training courses focusing on communication or researching best practice from leading authorities in this area are useful ways of advancing your knowledge. Some basic ideas are shared below to help you get started.

- **Be clear and concise with your instructions.** Avoid overly complex instructions and instead offer shorter instructions that scaffold the tasks you have planned for patients. Be clear and check back that patients understand what you have asked. Be ready to adapt the task you have planned if this is useful for the patient. Remember that the patient should always be your focus and located at the centre of your practice as an artist and participant.

- **Have examples ready to share to demonstrate the task you have planned.** Demonstrating or "modelling" a task can be a useful visual way of representing your instructions in a visual form. Think about demonstrating the activity with another member of your team to help support your participant to understand how the activity works. This can also be a useful way of supporting your participants with some ideas they could try out for the task.

- **Use interactive and visual stimuli.** There are many advantages to working online, including the possibilities of interactive media that responds instantly to your ideas. This can be built by practitioners on Google Jamboards or through touch-based resources on supporting tablets that allow participants to directly interact with a workshop, for example, using polling tools built into online platforms to allow participants to vote on an idea.

- **Think about non-verbal communication.** It's important not to privilege verbal communication over non-verbal forms of communication. Think about how you might add visual representations of instructions or symbols or simply add gestures when you are speaking as ways to make your communication clearer and more accessible for your participants.

- **Consider what your participant can see on screen.** Think about what your participants can see when you are online on their screen. For example, participants will always see your expression, so it is important to make sure you maintain a positive expression and ensure you are listening. This will help to reassure the participant that they are engaging with you. If you are making another expression, this can seem off-putting or show disinterest, which can understandably be both confusing and discourage participants from taking part in your session. This isn't easy to do while you are using transmedia and takes a little practice, so we would suggest running trial workshops with your peers before you do anything in person to help you.

Be responsive, spontaneous and creative in your practice

Being responsive, spontaneous and creative in your practice is important to ensure you can respond to uncertainty and unexpected reactions or incidents that can occur from time to time in healthcare settings. To help you navigate these moments, it is important to do the following.

- **Be open to feedback and action what clinical staff advise you.** Remember that clinical staff who you work with are the experts and they will guide you towards best practice. There are sometimes clashes in methodology and approach that happen when the arts meet healthcare contexts, so it's important to find ways to reconcile differences to make the practice you offer most effective. Taking feedback is a key skill; sometimes it can be challenging, particularly when people from different fields give feedback in different ways that you may not be familiar with. Try to agree how to give and hear feedback before you start your projects. This will help you navigate later and establish clear expectations and boundaries between your project partners.
- **Be ready to adapt to meet the access needs of your participants.** Remember that the needs of your participants, particularly in hospitals but also in care homes, can change

suddenly so you need to listen and respond in accordance with clinical staff advice. It may sound like we are repeating this point to you in different ways, but it is really important to be responsive and responsible in this context to follow best practice. To be responsive, you will need to follow clinical staff advice and support for different elements of your practice.

- **Consider how you follow the ideas of your participants to understand the flow of the session.** Following the interests that participants share with you sounds simple, but it can be complex and it's important to be mindful that directions of interest and engagement can vary through the course of a session. Being able to adapt and change direction is an important skill, and one well worth practising in tester workshops to see how you feel about sudden changes of topic and how you follow new threads that are offered to you. Having a strong, positive team will help you with this navigation and enable you to feel confident to make the choice to change direction rather than staying with a topic that no longer interests your participants.

- **Ask questions if you are unsure about something.** We have learnt from our students on placement that it is important to have space and time to ask questions. Some questions may need to be asked and responded to during a session, which is why it is important to build this into your guidance for clinical in-person staff. Other questions may arise after a workshop as you reflect on what happened and what you learnt. It is essential to make sure you can address new questions by organising a debrief with your team and clinical staff representative(s) to talk through your reflections. Make sure this is built into the time you need for each session so that clinical staff are fully aware of the support you require and the time this will take out of their days. Here are some questions we use when we debrief a workshop as guidance for you, but of course it's important to tailor these questions to your own ideas and experience. You will notice that the questions aren't passive; they are about taking action to improve practice so that each workshop you design builds on the learning from the previous session. It is important that everyone has the opportunity to respond to each question. It is equally important that everyone listens to and supports one another with advice as appropriate. Establishing agreed team ground rules for your debrief is important. We would strongly suggest creating an agreement with your group about being respectful and non-judgemental and offering support and advice as and when requested to help each other to learn and progress.

1. How did the session go?
2. What worked well?
3. What challenges did you face and how will you address them for next time?
4. What did you learn?
5. How did the participants respond?
6. Were there any safeguarding issues?
7. What do we need to do in preparation for the next session?

- **Being creative is very important.** It's important to think about how you creatively work together with your patients, ensuring you are supporting each person to realise their artistic vision. Being creative isn't just about being artistic; it is also about being spontaneous in your approach to make sure that you adapt to the flow of the session and the needs of the patient you are working with in response to clinical guidance.

- **Make sure your practice is cognitively stimulating and engaging.** It is important that you manage the activities you are facilitating to ensure they are exciting, innovative, and engaging. It's important not to make assumptions about what your participants can and cannot do and instead focus on ways of adapting your own practice to enable your patient to take part in the way they prefer to engage. Making sure activities are cognitively stimulating is important for patients to break up the monotony of the ward. Think back to the zone of proximal development that we discussed in Chapter 3 to help your thinking here.

- **Be prepared for moments of practice that are unexpected.** Remember to put the patient first in your workshop and if you are asked to finish a session early, have an exit strategy ready to help you. Similarly, if you are asked to extend your workshop, have a range of extension tasks ready in case you need them. If you need to change ideas and change the direction of your workshop, try to prepare by using non-linear workshop planning to have a range of exercises, tools and ideas ready to apply as and when they are needed. This will help you to feel prepared and stay flexible in your approach.

Summary thoughts

We hope that this book provides inspiration to those interested in arts and health. It isn't written as a comprehensive guide to practice but rather a sharing of our learning and development of this new type of practice so far. We are both passionate about the possibilities of arts and health and excited to be part of the future to shape practitioners interested in the developing field of social prescription. The opportunities we have been afforded and have afforded each other through our model of collaboration have meant that we have been able to share knowledge together, use our artistic skills, develop dementia-friendly creative projects and support students to learn our practice. We hope that you find the creative ideas shared in this book useful starting points for you, whether you are a student learning about applied theatre in community contexts, a practitioner seeking ideas for responsive digital practice or a healthcare professional thinking about integrating creativity into dementia care. Wherever your passion for arts in health comes from, it all adds up to make a big difference.

References

Abraham, N. (2021a). Lewis Loyd and Dementia Care Team: Imperial's Got Talent Entry 2021. [Online] Available at: www.youtube.com/watch?v=ax0-Q49vYoo&feature=youtu.be [Accessed 15 May 2022].

Abraham, N. (2021b). The Pedagogy of Reciprocity in Digital Applied Theatre Practice: The Antithesis to Unjust Responses to the COVID-19 Pandemic that Have Devalued and Ignored the Rights and Lives of Older Adults Living with Dementia. *Welfare e Ergonomia*, 7(2), pp. 49–63.

Abraham, N. (2019). The Intuit: An Investigation into the Definitions, Applications and Possibilities Offered by Intuitive Applied Theatre Practice with Vulnerable Youth. *Applied Theatre Research*. 7(2), pp. 233–249.

Abraham, N. and Ruddock, V. (2021). Your Story Your Way. In: L. Postlethwaite, ed., *Treasury of Arts Activities*, *Vol. 2*. London: Baring Foundation, pp. 20–21.

Alzheimer's Society (2022). *What is Dementia?* [Online] Available at: www.alz.org/alzheimers-dementia/what-is-dementia [Accessed 24 January 2022].

Bowell, P. and Heap, B. (2013). *Planning Process Drama: Enriching Teaching and Learning*. London: Routledge.

Brooker, D. and Latham, I. (2016). *Person-Centred Dementia Care: Making Services Better with the VIPS Framework*, 2nd edn. London: Jessica Kingsley Publishers.

Brown, S. L. (2009). *Play: How it Shapes the Brain, Opens the Imagination, and Invigorates the Soul*. New York: Avery.

Calderón-Larrañaga, S., Milner, Y., Clinch, M., Greenhalgh, T. and Finer, S. (2021). Tensions and Opportunities in Social Prescribing. Developing a Framework to Facilitate its Implementation and Evaluation in Primary Care: A Realist Review. *BJGP Open*, 5(3). [Online] Available at: https://bjgpopen.org/content/5/3/BJGPO.2021.0017 [Accessed 25 May 2022].

Csikszentmihalyi, M. (1997). *Finding Flow: The Psychology of Engagement with Everyday Life*. New York: Basic Books.

Csikszentmihalyi, M. (2013). *Creativity: The Psychology of Discovery and Invention*. New York: Harper Perennial Press.

Doran, G. T. (1981). There's a S.M.A.R.T. Way to Write Management's Goals and Objectives. *Management Review*, 70(11), pp. 35–36.

Etherington, K. (2004). *Becoming a Reflexive Researcher: Using Our Selves in Research*. London: Jessica Kingsley Publishers.

Elleström, L. (2013). Adaptations within the Field of Media Transformations. In: J. Bruhn, A. Gjelsvik and F. Hanssen, eds., *Adaptation Studies: New Challenges, New Directions*. London: Bloomsbury.

Freebody, K., Balfour, M., Finneran, M. and Anderson, M. (edd) (2018). *Applied Theatre: Understanding Change*. Cham, Switzerland: Springer.

Gonzalez-DeHass, A. R. and Willems, P. P. (2012). *Theories in Educational Psychology: Concise Guide to Meaning and Practice*. Lanham, MD: R&L Education.

Hapenciuc, A. (2019). The Influence of the Russian Psychological Pedagogy (by L. S. Lev Vygotsky) Upon the Model of Education Curricular Design in the American Cultural Space. *International Journal of Social and Educational Innovation (IJSEIro)*, 6(12), pp. 14–19.

Hayes, J. and Povey, S. (2011). *The Creative Arts in Dementia Care: Practical Person-Centred Approaches and Ideas.* London: Jessica Kingsley Publishers.

Hepplewhite, K. (2021). *The Applied Theatre Artist: Responsivity and Expertise in Practice.* London: Palgrave Macmillan.

Hughes, J. and Nicholson, H. (eds.) (2015). *Critical Perspectives on Applied Theatre.* Cambridge: Cambridge University Press.

Kerr, D. (2009). Ethics of Applied Theatre. *South African Theatre Journal*, 23(10), pp. 177–187.

James, J., Knight, J., Cotton, B., Freyne, R., Pettit, J., Gilby, L., Dunne, T., Gerard, N. and Jones, J. (2017). *Excellent Dementia Care in Hospitals: A Guide to Support People with Dementia and Their Carers.* London: Jessica Kingsley Publishers.

Kitwood, T. (1997). *Dementia Reconsidered: The Person Comes First.* Maidenhead: Open University Press.

Lanier, J. (2018). *Dawn of the New Everything: A Journey through Virtual Reality.* London: Vintage.

Lavender, A. (2017). The Internet, Theatre, and Time: Transmediating the Theatron. *Contemporary Theatre Review*, 27(3), pp. 340–352.

Lubin, J. (2012). The "Occupy" Movement: Emerging Protest Forms and Contested Urban Spaces. *Berkeley Planning Journal*, 25(1), pp. 184–197. [Online] Available at: www.escholarship.org/content/qt5rb320n3/qt5rb320n3_noSplash_6400b7bc03a5ce583aec3c3df25c8032.pdf [Accessed 23 January 2022].

McCormick, S. (2017). *Applied Theatre: Creative Ageing.* London: Bloomsbury.

McFadden, S. and McFadden, J. (2011). *Aging Together: Dementia, Friendship, and Flourishing Communities.* Baltimore, MD: The Johns Hopkins University Press.

NHS England (2019). Universal Personalised Care: Implementing the Comprehensive Model. [Online] Available at: www.england. nhs.uk/wp-content/uploads/2019/01/universal-personalised-care.pdf [Accessed 21 September 2021].

Niemtus, Z. (2018). Should We Be Less Smart on Targets? [Online] Available at: www.tes.com/magazine/archived/should-we-be-less-smart-targets [Accessed 8 May 2022].

Prentki, T. and Abraham, N. (2020). *The Applied Theatre Reader*. London: Routledge.

Prentki, T. and Preston, S. (2009). *The Applied Theatre Reader*. London: Routledge.

Preston, S. (2016). *Applied Theatre: Facilitation: Pedagogies, Practices, Resistance*. London: Bloomsbury.

Rahman, S. (2020). *Essentials of Delirium: Everything You Really Need to Know for Working in Delirium Care*. London: Jessica Kingsley Publishers.

Rahman, S. and Howard, R. (2018). *Essentials of Dementia: Everything You Really Need to Know for Working in Dementia Care*. London: Jessica Kingsley Publishers.

Rowlands, J. (2008) *Questioning Empowerment: Working with Women in Honduuras*. Oxford: Oxfam.

Royal College of Nursing (2021). Frailty in Older People. [Online] Available at: www.rcn.org.uk/clinical-topics/older-people/frailty [Accessed 24 January 2022].

Vygotsky, L. S. (1978). *Mind in Society: The Development of Higher Psychological Processes*, eds. M.Cole, V. John-Steiner, S. Scribner and E. Souberman. Cambridge, MA: Harvard University Press.

Winter, T. (2015). Praise & Criticism SMART Goal-Setting Model. [Online] Available at: https://blog.dtssydney.com/praise-critic ism-smart-goal-setting-model [Accessed 8 May 2022].

Recommended further reading

Communication

Astell, A. J., Shoaran, S. and Ellis, M. P. (2022). Using Adaptive Interaction to Simplify Caregiver's Communication with People with Dementia Who Cannot Speak. *Frontiers in Communication*, 6. [Online] Available at: www.frontiersin.org/articles/10.3389/fcomm.2021.689439/full#:~:text=Adaptive%20Interaction%20is%20a%20simplified,the%20people%20they%20care%20for [Accessed 13 June 2020].

Moore, L. A. and Davis, B. (2002). Quilting Narrative: Using Repetition Techniques to Help Elderly Communicators. *Geriatric Nursing*, 23(5), pp. 262–266.

Warren, W. (2021). Preserved Consciousness in Alzheimer's Disease and Other Dementias: Caregiver Awareness and Communication Strategies. *Frontiers in Psychology*, 12. [Online] Available at: www.frontiersin.org/articles/10.3389/fpsyg.2021.790025/full [Accessed 13 June 2020].

Technology and dementia

Gaber, S., Nygård, L., Brorsson, A., Kottorp, A. and Malinowsky, C. (2019). Everyday Technologies and Public Space Participation among People With and Without Dementia. *Canadian Journal of Occupational Therapy. Revue canadienne d'ergotherapie*, 86(5), pp. 400–411.

Kenigsberg, P. A. et al. (2019). Assistive Technologies to Address Capabilities of People with Dementia: From Research to Practice. *Dementia (London, England)*, 18(4), pp. 1568–1595.

Luscombe, N., Morgan-Trimmer, S., Savage, S. and Allen, L. (2021). Digital Technologies to Support People Living with Dementia in the Care Home Setting to Engage in Meaningful Occupations: Protocol for a Scoping Review. *Systematic Reviews*, 10(1), pp. 1–8.

Shastri, K. et al. (2022). Working Towards Inclusion: Creating Technology for and with People Living with Mild Cognitive Impairment or Dementia Who Are Employed. *Dementia (London, England)*, 21(2), pp. 556–578.

Multi-sensory practice

Bourdon, E. and Belmin, J. (2021). Enriched Gardens Improve Cognition and Independence of Nursing Home Residents with Dementia: A Pilot Controlled Trial. *Alzheimer's Research & Therapy*, 13(1), pp. 1–9.

Mahboubinia, M., Dalvandi, A., Nourozi, K., Mahmoudi, N. Safavi, S. S. and Hosseinzadeh, S. (2012). The Effect of Multi-Sensory Stimulation (MSS) on Cognitive Disturbances and Quality of Life of Male Patients with Alzheimer's Disease. *Iranian Rehabilitation Journal*, 10(1), pp. 50–55.

Solé, C., Cifré, I, Celdrán, M., Gaspar, M. and Rodríquez, L. (2019). Contributions of Multi-Sensory Stimulation (SNOEZELEN) in Older People with Dementia. *Asociación INFAD Universidad de Extremadura* (International Association of Educational and development Psychology for Childhood, Elderly and Disabled People), 2(1), pp. 311–320.

Prins, A. J., Scherder, E. J. A., van Straten, A., Zwaagstra, Y. and Milders, M. V. (2020). Sensory Stimulation for Nursing-Home Residents: Systematic Review and Meta-Analysis of Its Effects on

Sleep Quality and Rest-Activity Rhythm in Dementia. *Dementia and Geriatric Cognitive Disorders*, 49(3), pp. 219–234.

Regan, J. et al. (2019). Individualised Sensory Intervention to Improve Quality of Life in People with Dementia and Their Companions (SENSE-Cog trial): Study Protocol for a Randomised Controlled Trial. *Trials*, 20(1), pp. 1–15.

Co-creativity

Cousins, E., Tischler, V., Garabedia, C. and Dening, T. (2019). Principles and Features to Define and Describe Arts Interventions for People with Dementia: A Qualitative Realist Study. *Arts & Health*, 11(3), pp. 202–218.

Fleetwood-Smith, R., Tischler, V. and Robson, D. (2021). Using Creative, Sensory and Embodied Research Methods When Working with People with Dementia: A Method Story. *Arts & Health: International Journal for Research, Policy & Practice*, pp. 1–17. DOI: 10.1080/17533015.2021.1974064.

Tischler, V., Howson-Griffiths, T., Hedd Jones, C. and Windle, G. (2020). Using Art for Public Engagement: Reflections on the Dementia and Imagination Project. *Arts & Health*, 12(3), pp. 270–277.

Tischler, V. (2019). The Roving Diagnostic Unit: Art, Madness, Fun and the Potential for Change. *Arts & Health*, 11(2), pp. 174–182.

Tischler, V. (2018). "It Takes Me into Another Dimension": An Evaluation of Mental Health-Themed Exhibitions in Outdoor Urban Areas. *Arts & Health*, 10(1), pp. 1–16.

Person-centred practice

Brady, A.-M. et al. (2017). Responsive Community Care for People with Dementia and Their Families: Evaluating a Person-Centred and Integrated Care Model. *International Journal of Integrated Care (IJIC)*, 17(5), pp. 1–2.

Mitchell, G., Dupuis, S. L., Kontos, P., Jonas-Simpson, C. and Gray, J. (2020). Disrupting Dehumanising and Intersecting Patterns of Modernity with a Relational Ethic of Caring. *International Practice Development Journal*, 10(1), pp. 1–15.

Glossary

Key terms and definitions

Ageism

Ageism is a type of prejudice where someone is discriminated against based on their age. This may mean assumptions are made about someone's ability to do something, for example, access something or contribute to something once they enter the later stages of their lives (see McCormick, 2017).

Applied theatre

Applied theatre is an umbrella term to describe a set of practices that share traits. For example, applied theatre practitioners usually work with communities who are underrepresented or marginalised using theatre as a tool for social change, advocacy and development. Applied theatre projects are often created with, performed for or produced by communities (see Prentki and Preston, 2009; Hughes and Nicholson, 2015; Prentki and Abraham, 2020).

Artefacts

Artefacts are objects, or in our case also digital items, that are created as an output from our workshops with patients to celebrate or commemorate their identities/stories.

Bespoke

Bespoke is a term used to describe the uniqueness of something; it could also be seen as a synonym for personalised or individual. For our purposes, we have used this term to describe an artefact created for a patient that reflects their personal stories.

Consent

It is essential to ask consent, or permission, to engage patients in activities. This is part of best practice and is repeatedly asked to ensure both the patient and staff are happy with their in non-medical interventions. Consent for engagement is sought by clinical staff as specialists ahead of all project workshops for our specific practice.

Delirium

Delirium is an acute state of confusion and disorientation (see Rahman, 2020).

Dementia

Dementia is an umbrella term for a set of diseases that cause a deterioration in memory and thinking processes that impact on daily life (see Alzheimer's Society, 2022; Rahan and Howard, 2018).

Digital

Digital refers to the use of software or electronic devices.

Frailty

Frailty is a term to describe a syndrome rather than an illness. It relates to natural ageing and other changes such as declining fitness, changes in immune system or other long-term conditions that can affect someone's ability to recover from an injury or illness (See Royal College of Nursing, 2021).

Horizontal team structure

Horizontal teams are non-hierarchical. They are also referred to as having a flat structure and are based on collaboration rather than allocating a management structure.

Hyperlink

A hyperlink is an electronic connection between text or images that, when activated, opens a webpage, document, e-mail or other electronic asset.

Intergenerational

Intergenerational practice is a type of interaction that takes place with at least two different generations of people.

Jamboards

Jamboards are interactive online whiteboards where you can add digital post-its and images and draw pictures. Jamboards are collaborative spaces that allow multiple people to add ideas to the same digital space.

Pandemic

A pandemic is a worldwide spread of an illness or disease affecting a large proportion of people. COVID-19 has been described as a pandemic because of the way it has affected the world population.

Person-centred

Person-centred is an approach to creating tailored, personalised approaches to practice to support the needs, interests and preferences of people living with dementia (see Kitwood, 1997; Brooker and Latham, 2016).

Play

Play is a type of interaction that is imaginative, fantastical, aspirational and exciting. It often centres around imaging something happening or a possibility previously unexplored that an individual or group of people would like to discover. Play has connotations of belonging to children but it is very important to enable play in adults, which is connected to wellbeing, creativity and problem-solving (see Brown, 2009).

Process drama

Process drama is a drama-in-education methodology that involves the teacher taking on a character and the students also taking on one or more roles to go on a shared educational adventure, for example, to work together to solve a problem, explore a time in history or undertake a quest of some sort (see Bowell and Heap, 2013).

Reciprocity

Reciprocity is an interaction of exchange between two or more people. For our purposes, it is about thinking reflexively, empathetically and responsively about the way we interact with participants. It is also connected to our approach to sharing stories and ideas to collaboratively co-create artefacts that celebrate the stories of our participants.

Reflection

Reflection is a term used to consider what happened in the past and to think about or review an event, situation or interaction to see what we can learn about what took place.

Reflexivity

Reflexivity is deeper than just reflection. It isn't thinking just about what happened and what we can learn, but considers how and why this happened. For our purposes we invite students to think about their own history, context and beliefs and how these may have impacted their actions, interactions with and reactions to participants in workshops in addition to what we can learn about this and how we may want to change our approach as a result if necessary (see Etherington, 2004).

Virtual reality

Virtual reality (VR) is a type of technology that immerses the viewer/audience member in footage or gaming software that happens all around them. For our purposes, we are not referring to interactive gaming VR but instead focusing on VR360. This is a type of filmed footage which is a bespoke immersive experience created to respond to patient requests for locations, experiences or adventures (see Lanier, 2018).

Index

Lightning Source UK Ltd.
Milton Keynes UK
UKHW021837140922
408864UK00004B/76